Health Literacy - Advances and Trends

Edited by Carlos Miguel Rios González

Published in London, United Kingdom

Health Literacy - Advances and Trends
http://dx.doi.org/10.5772/intechopen.102241
Edited by Carlos Miguel Rios González

Contributors
Ouedraogo Ismaila, Borlli Michel Jonas Some, Roland Benedikter, Gayo Diallo, Heinz Bonfadelli, Mangesh Jabade, Seyda Dundar Ege, Osman Hayran

First published in London, United Kingdom, 2023 by IntechOpen
IntechOpen is the global imprint of INTECHOPEN LIMITED, registered in England and Wales, registration number: 11086078, 5 Princes Gate Court, London, SW7 2QJ, United Kingdom

British Library Cataloguing-in-Publication Data
A catalogue record for this book is available from the British Library

Additional hard and PDF copies can be obtained from orders@intechopen.com

Health Literacy - Advances and Trends
Edited by Carlos Miguel Rios González
p. cm.
Print ISBN 978-1-80356-308-4
Online ISBN 978-1-80356-309-1
eBook (PDF) ISBN 978-1-80356-310-7

Meet the editor

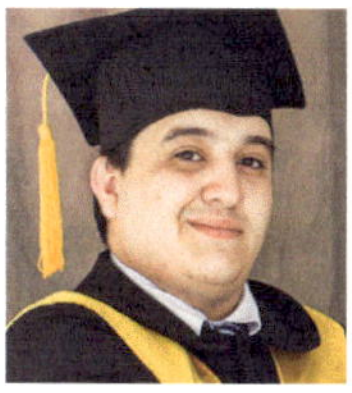

Carlos Miguel Rios González is a medical surgeon specializing in health research, university didactics, and infection control and hospital epidemiology. He is the Research Director at the Faculty of Medical Sciences, National University of Caaguazu, Paraguay. He is also a researcher and Director of Education at the National Institute of Health, Ministry of Public Health and Social Welfare, Director of the COCHRANE Paraguay Center, and president of Paraguay's Health Ethics Committee. He has a master's degree in hospital administration, a master's in scientific research methodology, a Ph.D. in public health and a Ph.D. in education, and is currently pursuing a master's in higher education in medical sciences. He is an editor and reviewer of international scientific journals as well as an international speaker.

Contents

Preface

The term "health literacy" began as a unique concept with its own frame of reference linked in one way or another to health education. Health literacy focuses on the individual and the information they receive and have available. The frame of reference for the development of health literacy is to be found in the Ottawa Charter for Health Promotion. In 2012, the European Consortium on Literacy for Health gave the following definition: "Literacy for health is linked to literacy and entails the knowledge, motivation and skills to access, understand and apply information on health issues, in order to make assessments and make decisions regarding daily health issues, disease prevention and health promotion, with the intention of maintaining or improving the quality of life in the course of this."

Health literacy is a fundamental public health tool that should be explored by the health systems of different countries, and encompasses two perspectives: clinical and public health. The clinical perspective includes elements that mainly reflect people's competencies within the healthcare environment, and the public health perspective includes dimensions beyond the healthcare environment, such as family, work and community.

This book contains five chapters. Chapter 1 discusses how to measure literacy, Chapter 2 considers the factors that influence it, Chapter 3 describes related technologies, Chapter 4 discusses the role of health professionals in organ donation, and Chapter 5 discusses how to measure literacy based on the importance of messages for self-management of chronic diseases

Health literacy is a fundamental tool of public health and should be explored by the health systems of different countries, for the improvement of public health.

Carlos Miguel Rios González
Facultad de Ciencias Médicas,
Universidad Nacional de Caaguazu,
Coronel Oviedo, Paraguay

Section 1

Advances

Chapter 1

How to Measure Organizational Health Literacy?

Osman Hayran and Seyda Dundar Ege

Abstract

Organizational Health Literacy (OHL) is defined as the ability of health organizations to provide services and information that are easy to find, understand and use, to assist people in decision making, and to remove existing barriers to all individuals who are seeking services. OHL is mainly related to communication, navigation, and leadership in organizations, which in turn leads to patient satisfaction, high quality of healthcare, better services for culturally diverse populations and people with disabilities, and risk minimization in healthcare services. Due to its multi-dimensional and complex nature, there are many criteria, ways, and methods for the implementation and evaluation of OHL. Although several measurement tools have been developed in the recent decade, valid and reliable scales are still needed to assess OHL levels in health care organizations. Brief information regarding these methods is presented in this section.

Keywords: organizational health literacy, healthcare organizations, assessment and evaluation, healthcare management, patient satisfaction

1. Introduction

Health literacy (HL) is an issue of increasing importance in the health sector due to its ability to use existing health services effectively and efficiently. It allows the acquisition of better outcomes from the services provided thus, reducing health expenditure. Study findings indicate that a significant number of successful results from health services are closely associated with the health literacy of individuals [1–3]. Its importance was better understood during the COVID-19 pandemic, because of the dependent relationship between individuals and the health care organizations.

The health literacy concept, which has been initially used to mean individuals' ability to read drug prospectuses, health-related brochures, and understand health-related information, has changed and expanded over time. Today, health literacy is defined as "people's knowledge, motivation, and competencies to access, understand, appraise, and apply health information to make judgments and take decisions in everyday life concerning healthcare, disease prevention, and health promotion to maintain or improve quality of life during the life course." [4], in essence, a lifelong learning activity that needs continuous improvement for individuals.

Over time, it has been understood that health literacy issue is not solely an individual burden, the health system and health organizations have an important role as well, so the "Organizational Health Literacy" (OHL) concept has been launched.

OHL is defined as the ability of health organizations to provide information and services that are easy to find, understand and use, to assist people in decision making, and to remove existing barriers to all individuals who are seeking services. Health literate health care organizations are organizations that provide the needed information and services to the people in an easier way of access, understanding, and use [5].

Literacy is not a genetic or an ordinary characteristic of the people. It is a phenomenon that emerges and develops under the influence of several variables. It is the product of a kind of interaction and that means there is a mutual and reciprocal action. For such action there must be at least two sides, a receiver and a sender or influencer. Additionally, it always occurs in an environment that has physical, social, and psychological characteristics. So, all of these variables regarding receiver, sender, and environment should be considered to understand the concept. That means health literacy is a product of an interaction between health-seeking individuals and the health care providers within the environment of health care organizations [6, 7].

Because measurement and evaluation methods of a feature is closely linked to its conceptualization, the concepts of HL and OHL should be clarified before discussing the measurement methods.

2. Health literacy (HL) and organizational health literacy (OHL)

The first use of the term health literacy was in the 1970s, during the times when health education was seen as a component of social policy, [8] and evolved in recent years. HL is expressed as the knowledge of individuals throughout their life course, which will guide behaviors and decisions related to themselves and public health, their knowledge of basic health information and services, their access to this information, their understanding of the information accessed, and then their use of this information for the development of health for the maintenance or improvement of quality of life. It is the degree to which individuals have the capacity to access, understand and interpret the basic health information, and services they need to make appropriate decisions associated with their health [4, 6].

Studies have reported that there is an association between low health literacy and various negative health behaviors as well as poor health-related outcomes, such as difficulties to interpret health messages and labels, poor medication adherence, high rates of hospitalization [9], frequent emergency room use, less frequent mammography rates [10], lower participation in preventive activities [11], inappropriate drug use, poor self-management of chronic conditions [12], high mortality rates [13], and increased health care costs [1, 14, 15].

Several definitions of health literacy [4, 16], as well as health literacy measures, were reported in different studies [15]. It is seen that more than 150 health literacy instruments were developed and used in the first decade of the 21st century according to various publications [17, 18].

Presence of different health literacy definitions and use of different measurement tools may be considered normal since they focus on different aspects of the concept and are complementary to each other. Here, the important thing to remember is that methods needed to measure health literacy are usually developed according to our understanding and definition of health literacy. In their study, Urstad et al. [15] have concluded that there will be a risk of missing information when the used measurement tools of health literacy are not consistent with the definition and concept of health literacy.

On the other hand, current health care systems have a complex nature and they are in rapid change and evolution. They usually are not designed according to the abilities of at least some of their service users and this characteristic makes it difficult for some patients to access and use the correct health information they needed. So, such systems should also be literate to help and increase the low literacy level of all patients.

The term OHL is relatively a new concept that emerged a few decades ago to address the challenges faced by individuals with predominantly limited HL. Because the service relationship in healthcare institutions and organizations is a mutual interaction, the literacy of institutions has become an important issue in recent years.

Features of the health organizations, such as a respectful approach to patients, easy access to services, easy information to understand, helpful navigation and signage systems, and correct answers given to every kind of question are important factors. These features are helpful to individuals for the correct use of the services, and they are as effective as the literacy of the individuals [5, 19, 20].

There are numerous studies showing that the development of OHL leads to positive effects on the health of patients and increases patient satisfaction [21–24]. Although there are various studies and ways on how an institution can become a health literate organization, agreed-upon methods to measure, and evaluate the level of OHL are still lacking. The existing methods are generally highly scoped, but their reliability and criterion validity are generally unknown since they are not used in interventional research.

3. Different approaches to measure OHL: conceptualization, implementation, and evaluation

OHL standards and measurement methods have become an increasingly important topic in the last decade. Although there is a strong interest in OHL, majority of the studies are theoretical, and methodological studies are limited. Presence of measurement methods with different characteristics causes confusion over OHL.

A recent review showed that at least 17 different measures were used to assess OHL. According to the findings of this scoping review, six major categories of OHL have been defined and the most prevalent topic is referred to as "communication with service users."

The following categories were, "easy access and navigation," "integration and prioritization of OHL," "assessments and organizational development," "engagement support of service users," and "information and qualification of staff" [25]. However, it was stated that no consensus has been reached on criteria that can describe a health care organization as a health literate organization.

Some criteria are focused on specific health facilities [26] or different aspects of OHL [26, 27] and/or interventions [26, 28], their evaluation [29] and implementation [30].

Another scoping review regarding OHL implementation has found that important factors that can be helpful for creating health literate organizations are ordered as, supportive leadership, a culture of change and innovation, awareness and participation of the staff, and engagement of service users [31]. However, different studies have also commented that still there is not a sufficient amount of evidence to assess the effects of OHL interventions on improved health outcomes or cost-effectiveness, and further studies are needed [26, 28].

As it was stated by Kaper et al. [31], interventional studies regarding the improvement of OHL have several weaknesses and the main limitations of the studies were lack of an experimental design and lack of instruments measuring OHL outcomes with known reliability and validity. Studies were usually conducted on small sample groups and without a control group or based on baseline cross-sectional measurements. Nevertheless, it is concluded that the instruments used in these studies may be useful to observe and monitor the change over time and make comparisons between the organizations [31].

Following are the most frequently referred studies regarding the conceptualization, implementation, and measures of the OHL.

3.1 Ten attributes of health literate health care organizations

The idea of a **health literate health care organization** (HLHCO) was introduced by the National Academy of Medicine of the USA in 2012. It is based on the concept developed by Schilinger and Keller [32]. The main principle of this concept is that every organization in the health system has to create an environment to promote easy access to all kinds of health information and services, better communication, and effective use of health services [7].

The comprehensive study, prepared by Brach et al. in 2012 [5], is a milestone in OHL. In this study, detailed recommendations on what health literate organizations should and should not be are clearly stated and Ten Attributes of Health Literate Health Care Organizations are defined.

Ten attributes of Health Literate Health Care Organizations are as follows [5]:

1. Has leadership that makes health literacy integral to its mission, structure, and operations.
   Health literacy is an organizational value for a health literate organization, and strategies of health literacy are internalized at every management level. They are perceived as part of the business and integral to its mission, structure, and operations. Leadership is the key to the success and sustainability of such an implementation.

2. Integrates health literacy into planning, evaluation measures, patient safety, and quality improvement.
   Health literacy is integrated into the strategic and operational plans of a health literate organization. It is seen as an inseparable part of patient safety and quality improvement activities and is evaluated regularly.

3. Prepares the workforce to be health literate and monitors progress.
   Every professional in the organization must be health literate and understand the meaning of being a health literate organization. So, they must be trained and educated by appropriate adult education methods for the establishment of a health literate organizational culture. Training and education activities must be continuous and monitored regularly. They must be organized under the responsibility of a training team and include every staff member.

4. Includes populations served in the design, implementation, and evaluation of health information and services.
   Community participation and decision sharing are essential for the success of all health care activities including health literacy. Health literate organizations include representatives of the local people in the design, implementation, and

evaluation of services. Especially hearing the voices of individuals with low health literacy is important for designing user-friendly services.

5. Meets the needs of populations with a range of health literacy skills while avoiding stigmatization.
   Health literate organizations use communication methods that are as simple as possible. Written, visual or digital communication is not sufficient since some individuals may have difficulties. So, alternatives such as oral communication and escort guiding are useful methods. These methods must be available for and offered to every service user to reduce the low literacy-related stigma. This is particularly important for individuals who have limited health literacy.

6. Uses health literacy strategies in interpersonal communications and confirms understanding at all points of contact.
   Health literate organizations create an environment that has linguistic and cultural competency to support health literacy strategies. Such an environment aims to provide clear communication during all interactions and for every kind of service including clinical, administrative, and financial services.

7. Provides easy access to health information and services and navigation assistance.
   Health literate organizations design their facilities to help people to access information and services easily. They use a simple and easy-to-understand style of symbols, language, and signage.

8. Designs and distributes print, audiovisual, and social media content that is easy to understand and act on.
   Health literate organizations design all printed materials, such as education documents, diagnosis and treatment guides, laboratory test results, insurance policies, bills, and various written directives in an understandable style and with easy-to-understand language. The same approach is true for the design and distribution of audiovisual and social media content.

9. Addresses health literacy in high-risk situations, including care transitions and communications about medicines.
   "First, do no harm" is the number one principle of medicine since Hippocrates. However, due to the nature of the health services, there are several high-risk situations that cannot be eradicated in health facilities. Complications following surgical operations, adverse drug reactions, and absence of radical therapies are some examples of these situations. Health literate health care organizations identify such situations and inform patients appropriately.

10. Communicates clearly what health plans cover and what individuals will have to pay for services.

Health literate organizations communicate openly, clearly, and on time regarding financial issues such as coverage of the patient's health plans, and how much they will have to pay for which services. They answer all relevant questions of the service users in an understandable language.

The ten attributes are related to health organizations, health care professionals, and various types of healthcare facilities that have direct responsibility for the provision of health services. All kinds of hospitals, clinics, group practices, private physician offices, community health centers, pharmacies, health insurance companies, accreditation agencies, information technology and health education professionals, and administrative staff needed to have these attributes to become health literate. In other words, almost all components of the supply side of a health system must have these ten attributes.

"Ten attributes of health literate healthcare organization" has been used by many researchers in the following years.

In a study conducted by Kowalski et al. [33] a ten items survey tool "Health Literate Health Care Organization Ten Item Questionnaire" (HLHO-10) to represent the ten attributes was developed. It was applied as part of a larger study and cross-sectional data was collected from a key informant survey in 51 German hospitals, and found to be reliable and valid [33]. It was concluded to be a useful tool to assess the level of OHL that is which organizations are helpful to their users to access, find, understand, and use the correct information they needed as well as the services.

Later HLHO-10 has been used during a survey to assess the OHL of a group of hospitals in Turkey and investigate the relationships between OHL, patient satisfaction, and individual health literacy by Hayran and Ozer [21].

Bonaccorsi et al., have used the Italian version of the HLHO-10 scale in healthcare organizations in Tuscany. They have found that accredited hospitals have higher HLHO-10 scores and perceived quality increases with the increase in HLHO-10 scores, which is interpreted as OHL an integral element for the quality of care [34].

HLHO-10 scale was also adapted to measure and use the OHL level of the facilities established for individuals with various disabilities [35].

Ten attributes provided intellectual foundation to other action frameworks. At least two other concepts and tools were based on the principles of the ten attributes. These are, "Vienna Concept of Health Literate Hospitals and Healthcare Organizations" (V-HLO) [36] and "the Organizational Health Literacy Responsiveness self-assessment tool" (Org-HLR) [37].

3.2 V-HLO

(Vienna Concept of Health Literate Hospitals and Healthcare Organizations)

V-HLO is designed as a self-assessment questionnaire that includes 9 standards, 22 sub-standards, and 160 items [36]. It was tested by Pelikan and Dietscher in Austria and found to be successful [38].

This tool builds upon the "Ten Attributes of Health Literate Health Care Organizations." However, the V-HLO expands the concept by introducing specific aspects tested in Health Promoting Hospitals (HPH) that were created by an international working group within the 'International Network of Health Promoting Hospitals. It includes five standards published by WHO-EURO [39], 18 strategies of the HPH [40], and with reference to quality management concepts.

V-HLO considers the significance of organizational support for health literacy as a necessary precondition for sustainable implementation. This support is necessary for the implementation of interventions in relation to four action areas of the concept. These action areas are health literacy that is needed to gain adequate **access to health care**, **to participate in treatment and care**, to take adequate **decisions and actions in relation to disease prevention and health promotion**, and also **lifestyle development**.

These action areas are applied to three stakeholder groups, namely, patients, staff, and population.

Nine standards of V-HLO are as follows [38]:

1. Establishment of management policy and organizational structures for health literacy (includes 2 sub-standards)

2. Development of materials and services in participation with stakeholders (includes 2 sub-standards)

3. Qualification of staff for health-literate communication with service users (includes 2 sub-standards)

4. Provision of a supportive environment with health-literate navigation and access (includes 5 sub-standards)

5. Application of health literacy principles in routine communication with patients (includes 4 sub-standards)

6. Improvement of the health literacy of patients and their entourage (includes 2 sub-standards)

7. Improvement of the health literacy of the staff (includes 2 sub-standards)

8. Contribution to the health literacy in the region (includes 2 sub-standards)

9. Sharing experiences and being a role model (includes 1 sub-standard)

In the following years, the French version of V-HLO has been prepared and tested in three hospitals in Belgium. It was concluded to be an appropriate tool for hospitals that have the intention to raise their level of health literacy, create awareness and formulate strategies and actions [41].

3.3 OHL Self-AsseT

(Self-Assessment Tool to Promote Organizational Health Literacy in Primary Care Settings)

OHL Self-AsseT is a self-assessment tool that was developed by De Ganni et al. to evaluate the level of OHL in primary health care settings in Switzerland [42].

The rationale underlying this Project was the need for a specific tool to assess and enhance OHL in primary health care settings. As the authors have stated, most approaches to OHL have usually focused on inpatient care, and outpatient and/or primary health care services have rarely been included. However, especially the level of OHL in primary care settings is of great importance, because they are the first contact points of the well-designed health systems.

The tool has been developed and evaluated with the participation of various practice partners including general practitioners and community health care organizations as well as expert opinions. The aim of this tool is to make the needs assessment, identify the improvement areas, and implement the actions necessary for OHL.

The tool consists of three modules and six dimensions:

- A user manual containing instructions

- A checklist for self-assessment of the community health services
- A handbook to measure the improvement of the check-list items

Six dimensions of the tool were based on the ten attributes of a health literate health care organization [5], the nine standards of the V-HLO [38], and six dimensions of a health literate organization as used in the Tasmanian toolkit [HelloTAS] [43] and finalized after discussions with the representatives of primary care professionals the community health care organizations.

Six dimensions of the tool included the main content of the checklist. Then it was divided into 15 sub-dimensions including a total of 43 criteria (**Table 1**).

Authors have concluded that this tool may be helpful for a successful implementation of OHL in primary care settings because it was developed with the participation of various practice partners and shaped by expert opinions.

3.4 Org-HLR tool

(Development of the Organizational Health Literacy Responsiveness self-assessment tool and process)

In their study, Trezona et al. [37] developed the Organizational Health Literacy Responsiveness self-assessment tool (Org-HLR) and conducted an assessment process for supporting the health organizations with the application of the tool.

OHL responsiveness is the synonym term for OHL. It means the provision of health information and services in an equitable manner in terms of access and participation, taking into consideration the literacy needs and preferences of all service

Dimensions	Sub-dimensions (number of criteria)
1. Provision of easy access to primary care services and facilitated navigation	1.1 Contact (5) 1.2 Navigation within the primary care service (2)
2. Communication in plain and easy to understand language	2.1 Oral communication (8) 2.2 Written communication (5)
3. Promotion of health literacy for service users	3.1 Empowering service users to use health information (1) 3.2 Promotion of an active role and self-management of service users (2)
4. Promotion of health literacy of staff members	4.1 Know-how and professional competence (1) 4.2 Personnel development (3) 4.3 Staff members' health (1)
5. Incorporation of health literacy into management and organizational structure	5.1 Health literacy as an organizational responsibility (2) 5.2 Health literacy as a development goal (2) 5.3 Organizational culture (2) 5.4 User involvement – feedback (2)
6. Promotion of health literacy at care interfaces, networks, and further activities of the organization	6.1 Care interfaces (4) 6.2 Networking and further activities (3)

Adapted from De Ganni et al. [42].

Table 1.
"Organizational Health Literacy Self-Assessment Tool for Primary Care" (OHL self-AsseT).

users, and supporting community participation during decision-making processes for health and well-being [37].

The self-rating Org-HLR tool and process were derived through co-design processes with a wide range of professionals working in the health and social services sectors, It has seven dimensions for assessment and they are divided into 24 sub-dimensions with 135 performance indicators.

Seven assessment dimensions are:

1. External policy and funding environment

2. Leadership and culture

3. Systems, processes, and policies

4. Access to services and programs

5. Community engagement and partnerships

6. Communication practices and standards

7. Workforce

3.5 OHL-Hosp

(Rating Scale for Secondary and Tertiary Care Hospitals)

A scale to assess the OHL status of different types of secondary and tertiary care hospitals has been developed by Dundar Ege and Hayran [44]. Forty-three 7-point Likert-type scale items were prepared by a comprehensive literature review and shaped by expert opinions. It was tested by the management staff of a sample group of 47 hospitals in İstanbul, including State hospitals, Private Hospitals, University Hospitals, Non-Profit Foundation Hospitals, and Accredited and Non-accredited Hospitals.

Five dimensions of OHL-Hosp were identified following the exploratory and confirmatory factor analyses. Internal consistency of the items of each dimension has been found significantly high and statistically significant (**Table 2**).

The scale consisting of 43 items and five dimensions is concluded to be a valid and reliable instrument to determine OHL levels of secondary and tertiary care institutions.

Dimensions (number of items)	Eigenvalues	Variance (%)	Cronbach's alpha
1. Leadership and Regulations (16)	20.996	48.828	0.987
2. Communication (14)	5.014	11.661	0.946
3. Operational Access (6)	3.320	7.722	0.954
4. Indoor Access (4)	2.973	6.914	0.948
5. Outdoor Access (3)	1.638	3.810	0.841

Table 2.
Dimensions and factor analysis findings of the OHL-Hosp scale.

3.6 The HLE2 assessment tool

(Health Literacy Environment of Hospitals and Health Centers: Access to Information, Care, and Services Through the Lens of Health Literacy)

This tool is the updated version of the "Health Literacy Environment of Hospitals and Health Centers" by Rudd and Andersen [45]. It was developed by Harvard University and published in 2019 [7]. Its original form has been widely used in the USA. It was also adapted to use in different countries including Australia, New Zealand and European countries.

It is helpful to identify and rate the factors that are related to the literacy of health organizations for improving health literacy and monitoring change over time.

The HLE2 tool is organized into five sections, 10 parts, and 135 criteria as it is presented in **Table 3**. Content of all sections is addressed through the lens of health literacy. Each section has a rating scale. Following data collection, a total score and a percentage score is computed for each section. An overall score tally of the HLE2 has not been recommended. Instead, actions to consider for the % score of each section are described.

The study is based on visitor observations and standards to be applied by officials and it is organized as a list of things to do for OHL. The list can be applied in the form of brainstorming sessions with active members of healthcare institutions.

3.7 Findings from comprehensive literature reviews

3.7.1 The work of Bremer et al.

In a scoping review [25] which was held in 2021, sixty studies on OHL are examined in-depth and common six main categories, 25 subcategories of attributes, and 494 criteria of OHL were identified.

The main categories were ordered as:

- Communication with service users

Sections	Parts (number of criteria)
1. Organizational Policies	• Part 1 focuses on policies in written format (6) • Part 2 focuses on policies on practice (6)
2. Organizational Practices	• Part 1 focuses on institutional resources (5) • Part 2 focuses on orientation, development, and expectations (15)
3. Navigation	• Part 1 focuses on arrival (10) • Part 2 focuses on wayfinding (19)
4. Culture and Language	(10)
5. Communication	• Part 1 focuses on Print Materials (20 items) • Part 2 focuses on Forms (12 items) • Part 3 focuses on Web Postings (18 items) • Part 4 focuses on Patient Portals (14 items)

Adapted from "HLE2" [7].

Table 3.
The HLE2 assessment tool

- Easy access and navigation
- Integration and prioritization
- Assessments and organizational development
- Engagement and support of service users
- Information and qualification of staff

Among the reviewed articles published between 2006 and 2020, the majority were related to toolkits. This was followed by discussions, case studies, feasibility studies, surveys, workshop summaries, or evaluation studies.

"Ten Attributes of Health Literate Health Care Organizations" by Brach et al. [5] was the most frequently referred publication for the concepts used.

Reviewed studies have used 17 different assessment tools and instruments for the assessment of OHL. The HLHO-10 [33] and the HLE2 [7, 45] were the most frequently referenced tools among them.

The tools were usually designed as questionnaires and used during surveys. Some studies have used them in their original form while others have used a subset of items. Some studies have used the translated tools in a different language while others have adopted the measures for a different type of method.

Design of the assessment methods has also varied. Some studies have used standardized questionnaires and semi-structured interviews while others have collected the data by observations, checklists, and material assessments.

However, the authors have stated that the majority of the tools and instruments were not tested for validity and feasibility.

3.7.2 The work of Brega et al.

The goal of the study was to develop a valuable set of measures to inform OHL-related quality improvement activities. The study [46] was based on patient feedback and presented the standards that increase quality in healthcare organizations.

These are organizational structure, policy and leadership, communication, navigation, and patient participation. The results are similar to other studies.

3.7.3 The work of Lubash et al.

Communication has been deeply examined as the main standard of OHL in this study in 2021 [47]. A sensitive communication approach was assessed from the perspective of the patients' health in complex care structures.

As an important finding of the study, better processing of the organization is perceived by patients that was related to significantly higher health literacy scores. On the other hand, better health literacy scores were related to more patient-reported social support provided by physicians and nurses as well as fewer unmet information needs.

It was concluded that investing in good processing of the organization can improve the communication that is sensitive to health literacy. This has the potential to encourage service user–provider relationships and it might reduce the unmet information needs of the service users.

3.7.4 The work of Farmanova et al.

In this meta-narrative review, Farmanova et al. have identified 20 health literacy guides with various contexts and scopes [27]. Most guides have been prepared for general healthcare organizations. Six of them were specific for primary care besides hospitals and pharmacies. One was specific to health literacy of nursing practices.

Most included dimensions of OHL in guides were verbal and written communication, and access and navigation. All guides have included these dimensions. Access and navigation referred to the physical environment as well as the provided services by the organization.

Thirteen key barriers under 3 broad themes were identified during the use of health literacy guides: barriers related to the leadership and cultural environment of the organization; barriers related to the design and planning of interventions needed for the improvement; and barriers referred to the health workforce.

Especially recent guides provided best practices and recommendations that are evidence-based to support OHL actions. However, it was found that most of the guides have not been tested and their applicability was unknown in organizational practices, and this finding raises questions regarding their effectiveness [27].

Authors have concluded that OHL seems to be a heterogeneous phenomenon and it can be theorized from many different perspectives and implemented in different ways.

4. Conclusions

There is a similarity among the criteria identified in the conceptualization of the OHL in various studies. However, despite the conceptual similarities and presence of many different techniques and scales to assess OHL, there is still confusion about conceptualization and operationalization [25].

"Ten Attributes of Health Literate Organizations" by Brach et al. [5], is the most detailed and broad-ranged study in terms of conceptualization of OHL and has been an intellectual foundation for several other studies. Many of the assessment tools and instruments were based on the principles described as ten attributes. Most frequently used examples are, HLHO-10 [33], V-HLO [36], and the Org-HLR [37].

HLHO-10 is designed as a questionnaire that rates each of the ten attributes on a Likert scale.

The V-HLO aims at the sustainability of OHL and expands the concept by introducing specific aspects tested in Health Promoting Hospitals (HPH) [39, 40]. It approaches OHL from the stakeholders' view considering their impact zone.

The Org-HLR uses health literacy responsiveness as a system-level action. It aims to coordinate and integrate all health care services, and system navigation by intersectoral collaboration [37].

Another important instrument HLE2 Assessment Tool [7] has a long history and wider use and includes palpable criteria mostly based on observations regarding implementation details. It offers 'to-do lists', observation forms, and process management details that can also be used during brainstorming meetings in organizations.

Among the several criteria to describe OHL, "communication" seems to be the major and most common component in all studies. Possible benefit effects of HL-sensitive communication were examined in several studies [47] including specific groups such as cancer patients [48], culturally diverse patient groups [49], and concluded to be an important dimension of OHL.

"Ease of access and navigation" is another significant criterion to describe OHL that has been investigated in many studies. Zanobi et al. [26] and Bremer et al. [25] have identified many different interventions for easy access and navigation in their scoping reviews. Use of pathways with different color codes, directions prepared with a plain and standardized language, support from volunteer escorts, directions posted in commonly used languages, and navigation apps are some examples. However, no studies have been found to evaluate their effects.

In some studies, quality is considered the main aspect [46] and OHL is examined as an instrument to raise the quality of healthcare.

It is known that patient satisfaction and responsiveness are high in organizations with high OHL [21]; however, it is not possible to say the opposite and it is important not to confuse OHL with patient satisfaction or health care responsiveness.

According to a study conducted during the COVID-19 pandemic, OHL principles and guidelines may be helpful to promote human-centered health care and services even in times of crisis [50].

OHL has been examined in various countries, in different settings, and from different aspects by many researchers. Among the limited number of scales that have been presented in some studies, none of them was tested for validity and reliability [51].

Additionally, many patient health outcomes have been investigated, but it is seen that almost all of them were related to supportive interventions for patients. No study was found reporting the patient health outcomes that are related to staff.

The effects of environmental support on health care staff have been rarely studied. Only a few studies have reported outcomes related to the satisfaction and helpfulness perception of the staff [26].

Comprehensive work done by Brach et al. on the conceptualization of the OHL is a milestone as we have mentioned above [5]. It serves as an intellectual base for other studies. In studies, regarding the implementation and assessment of OHL, checklists based on on-site observation and interview forms based on general questions for qualitative evaluation purposes are used. Furthermore, in some studies, it is observed that checklists for self-evaluation and guidelines to assess the healthcare organizations including primary healthcare institutions are also used.

In a comprehensive systematic review, it was found that the practices, measurement, and evaluation criteria in the field of OHL are very diverse and differ from each other [52]. According to the results of the screening, there were 8 main measurement-evaluation tools used for OHL measurement-evaluation, among which HLHO-10 (Health Literate Health Organization-10) [33] and V-HLO (Vienna Health Literate Organization) [36, 38] were used more frequently.

No definitive list of actions for implementation was found as well as assessment and measurement of the OHL. As a matter of fact, the rapid change in health care systems, institutions, types of services, technologies, and even professions naturally will affect and change the ways of our understanding of OHL.

So, aims for the implementation, operationalization, and improvement of the OHL must be addressed in a systematic and flexible manner. This issue is particularly significant for the communication of health care organizations with service users.

As the last word, some recommended steps to facilitate organizational change when promoting OHL practices can be summarized as encouragement of leadership, presence of clear and effectively communicated change vision, and provision of staff training and education to promote OHL practices [53]. These are the most important steps during the journey to facilitate organizational change toward OHL.

Author details

Osman Hayran* and Seyda Dundar Ege
Istanbul Medipol University, Istanbul, Turkey

*Address all correspondence to: ohayran@gmail.com

References

[1] Berkman N, Sheridan S, Donahue K, Halpern D, Crott K. Low health literacy and health outcomes: An updated systematic review. Annals of Internal Medicine. 2011;**155**(2):97-107. DOI: 10.7326/0003-4819-155-2-201107190-00005

[2] Charet GP. Hospitals address health literacy for improved care, cost savings. Hospitals and Health Networks. 2010;**85**(5):14 PMID: 20578307

[3] Eichler K, Wieser S, Brügger U. The costs of limited health literacy: A systematic review. International Journal of Public Health. 2009;**54**:313-324. DOI: 10.1007/s00038-009-0058-2

[4] Sorensen K, Van den Broucke S, Fullam J, Doyle G, Pelican J, Slonska Z, et al. Health literacy and public health: A systematic review and integration of definitions and models. BMC Public Health. 2012;**12**(1):80. DOI: 10.1186/1471-2458-12-80

[5] Brach C, Keller D, Hernandez LM, Baur C, Parker R, Dreyer B, et al. Ten Attributes of Health Literate Health Care Organizations. NAM Perspectives, Discussion Paper. Washington, DC: National Academy of Medicine; 2012. DOI: 10.31478/201206a

[6] Institute of Medicine (IOM). Health Literacy: A Prescription to End Confusion. Washington DC: The National Academies Press; 2004. pp. 1-16

[7] Rudd RE, Oelschlegel S, Grabeel KL, Tester E, Heidel E. The HLE2 Assessment Tool. Boston: Harvard T.H. Chan School of Public Health; 2019. Available from: https://cdn1.sph.harvard.edu/wp-content/uploads/sites/135/2019/05/april-30-FINAL_The-Health-Literacy-Environment2_Locked.pdf [Accessed: May 5, 2022]

[8] Simonds SK. Health education as social policy. Health Education Monographs. 1974;**2**(1_suppl):1-10. DOI: 10.1177/10901981740020S102

[9] Mitchell SE, Sadikova E, Jack BW, et al. Health literacy and 30-day postdischarge hospital utilization. Journal of Health Communication. 2012;**17**:325-338

[10] O'Hara J, McPhee C, Dodson S, et al. Barriers to breast cancer screening among diverse cultural groups in Melbourne, Australia. International Journal of Environmental Research and Public Health. 2018;**15**:1677

[11] Chen J-Z, Hsu H-C, Tung H-J, et al. Effects of health literacy to self-efficacy and preventive care utilization among older adults. Geriatrics & Gerontology International. 2013;**13**:70-76

[12] Olesen K, Reynheim AL, Joensen L, et al. Higher health literacy is associated with better glycemic control in adults with type 1 diabetes: A cohort study among 1399 Danes. BMJ Open Diabetes Research & Care. 2017;**5**:e000437

[13] Bostock S, Steptoe A. Association between low functional health literacy and mortality in older adults: Longitudinal cohort study. BMJ. 2012;**344**:e1602

[14] Kickbusch I, Pelikan JM, Apfel F, Tsouro AD. Health Literacy. The Solid Facts. Geneva: World Health Organization; 2013

[15] Urstad KH, Andersen MH, Larsen MH, et al. Definitions and

measurement of health literacy in health and medicine research: A systematic review. BMJ Open. 2022;**12**:e056294. DOI: 10.1136/bmjopen-2021-056294

[16] Liu C, Wang D, Liu C, et al. What is the meaning of health literacy? A systematic review and qualitative synthesis. Family Medicine and Community Health. 2020;**8**:e000351

[17] O Neill B, Gonçalves D, Ricci-Cabello I, et al. An overview of self-administered health literacy instruments. PLoS One. 2014;**9**:e109110

[18] Haun JN, Valerio MA, McCormack LA, et al. Health literacy measurement: An inventory and descriptive summary of 51 instruments. Journal of Health Communication. 2014;**19**:302-333

[19] Koh HK, Berwick DM, Clancy CM, Baur C, Brach C, Harris LM, et al. New Federal Policy Initiatives to boost health literacy can help the nation move beyond the cycle of costly crisis care. Health Affairs. 2012;**31**(2):434-443. DOI: 10.1377%2Fhlthaff.2011.1169

[20] Koh HK, Brach C, Harris LM, Parchman ML. A proposed 'health literate care model would constitute a systems approach to improving patients' engagement in care. Health Affairs. 2013;**32**(2):357-367. DOI: 10.1377%2Fhlthaff.2012.1205

[21] Hayran O, Ozer O. Organizational health literacy as a determinant of patient satisfaction. Public Health. 2018;**163**:20-26. DOI: 10.1016/j.puhe.2018.06.011

[22] Jukkala A, Deupree JP, Graham S. Knowledge of limited health literacy at an academic health Center. Journal of Continuing Education in Nursing. 2009;**40**:298-302. DOI: 10.3928/00220124-20090623-01

[23] Groene OR, Rudd R. Results of a feasibility study to assess the health literacy environment: Navigation, written and Oral communication in ten hospitals in Catalonia, Spain. Journal of Communication in Healthcare. 2011;**4**:227-237. DOI: 10.1179/1753807611Y.0000000005

[24] Weaver NL, Wray RJ, Zellin S, Gautam K, Jupka K. Advancing organizational health literacy in healthcare organizations serving high-needs populations: A case study. Journal of Health Communication. 2012;**17**:55-66. DOI: 10.1080/10810730.2012.714442

[25] Bremer D, Klockmann I, Jaß L, Härter M, von dem Knesebeck O, Lüdecke D. Which criteria characterize a health literate healthcare organization? – A scoping review on organizational health literacy. BMC Health Services Research. 2021;**21**(664):2-14. DOI: 10.1186/s12913-021-06604-z

[26] Zanobini P, Lorini C, Baldasseroni A, Dellisanti C, Bonaccorsi G. A scoping review on how to make hospitals health literate healthcare organizations. International Journal of Environmental Research and Public Health. 2020;**17**(3):1036. DOI: 10.3390/ijerph17031036

[27] Farmanova E, Bonneville L, Bouchard L. Organizational health literacy: Review of theories, frameworks, guides, and implementation issues. Inquiry. 2018;**55**:46958018757848. DOI: 10.1177/0046958018757848

[28] Lloyd JE, Song HJ, Dennis SM, Dunbar N, Harris E, Harris MF. A paucity of strategies for developing health literate organisations: A systematic review. PLoS One. 2018;**13**(4):e0195018. DOI: 10.1371/journal.pone.0195018

[29] Rowlands G, Trezona A, Russell S, Lopatina M, et al. What Is the Evidence on the Methods, Frameworks and

Indicators Used to Evaluate Health Literacy Policies, Programmes and Interventions at the Regional, National and Organizational Levels? Copenhagen: WHO Regional Office for Europe; 2019

[30] Palumbo R. Designing health-literate health care organization: A literatüre review. Health Services Management Research. 2016;**29**(3):79-87. DOI: 10.1177/0951484816639741

[31] Kaper MS, Sixsmith J, Reijneveld SA, de Winter AF. Outcomes and critical factors for successful implementation of organizational health literacy interventions: A scoping review. International Journal of Environmental Research and Public Health. 2021;**18**(22): 11906. DOI: 10.3390/ijerph182211906

[32] Schillinger D, Keller D. The Other Side of the Coin: Attributes of a Health Literate Healthcare Organization. Commissioned by the Institute of Medicine Roundtable on Health Literacy. In: IOM (Institute of Medicine). How Can Health Care Organizations Become More Health Literate?: Workshop Summary. Washington, DC: The National Academies Press, 2012. Available from: https://www.ncbi.nlm.nih.gov/books/NBK201219/; 2011

[33] Kowalski C, Lee SY, Schmidt A, Wesselmann S, Wirtz MA, Pfaff H, et al. The health literate health care organization 10 item questionnaire (HLHO-10): Development and validation. BMC Health Services Research. 2015;**15**:47. DOI: 10.1186/s12913-015-0707-5

[34] Bonaccorsi G, Romiti A, Ierardi F, Innocenti M, Del Riccio M, Frandi S, et al. Health-literate healthcare organizations and quality of Care in Hospitals: A cross-sectional study conducted in Tuscany. International Journal of Environmental Research and Public Health. 2020;**17**(7):2508. DOI: 10.3390/ijerph17072508

[35] Rathmann K, Vockert T, Wetzel LD, Lutz J, Dadaczynski K. Organizational health literacy in facilities for people with disabilities: First results of an explorative qualitative and quantitative study. International Journal of Environmental Research and Public Health. 2020;**17**(8):2886. DOI: 10.3390/ijerph17082886

[36] Dietscher C, Lorenc J, Pelikan JM. Pilottestung Zum "Selbstbewertungsinstrument für Die Organizationale Gesundheitskompetenz von Krankenhäusern" gemäß dem Wiener Konzept Gesundheitskompetenter Krankenbehandlungsorganisationen. [Piloting of the "Self-Assessment Tool to Investigate the Organizational Health Literacy of Hospitals" Following the Vienna Concept of a Health Literate Health Care Organization.]. Vienna: Ludwig Boltzmann Institute; 2015 Available from: http://www.ongkg.at/downloads-links/downloads.html

[37] Trezona A, Dodson S, Osborne RH. Development of the organizational health literacy responsiveness (org-HLR) self-assessment tool and process. BMC Health Services Research. 2018;**18**:694. DOI: 10.1186/s12913-018-3499-6

[38] Pelikan JM, Dietscher C. Health-literate hospitals and healthcare organizations. Results from an Austrian feasibility study on the self-assessment of organizational health literacy in hospitals. In: Schaeffer D, Pelikan JM, editors. Health Literacy: Forschungsstand Und Perspektiven [Health Literacy: Status of Research and Perspectives]. Bern: Hogrefe; 2016

[39] Groene O. Implementing Health Promotion in Hospitals. Manual and Self-Assessment Form. Copenhagen: World Health Organization; 2006

[40] Pelikan JM, Krajic K, Dietscher C. The health promoting hospital (HPH):

Concept and development. Patient Education and Counseling. 2001;**45**(4):239-243. DOI: 10.1016/s0738-3991(01)00187-2 PMID: 11755767

[41] Henrard G, Vanmeerbeek M, Dardenne N, Rademakers J. The Vienna self-assessment questionnaire: A usable tool towards more health-literate hospitals? Explorative case studies in three hospitals in Belgium. BMC Health Services Research. 2021;**21**(1):287. Published 2021 Mar 31. DOI: 10.1186/s12913-021-06211-y

[42] De Gani SM, Nowak-Flück D, Nicca D, Vogt D. Self-assessment tool to promote organizational health literacy in primary care settings in Switzerland. International Journal of Environmental Research and Public Health. 2020;**17**(24):9497. DOI: 10.3390/ijerph17249497

[43] HeLLo TAS! Available from: https://www.hellotas.org.au [Accessed: May 6, 2022]

[44] Ege ŞD, Hayran O. Scale development for organizational health literacy. ESTUDAM. 2022;**7**(2):243-256. DOI: 10.35232/estudamhsd.991545

[45] Rudd RE, Anderson JE. The Health Literacy Environment of Hospitals and Health Centers. Boston, MA: National Center for the Study of Adult Learning and Literacy (NCSALL); 2006. p. 153. Available from: https://eric.ed.gov/?id=ED508596 [Accessed: May 7, 2022]

[46] Brega AG, Hamer MK, Albright K, Brach C, Saliba D, Abbey D, et al. Organizational health literacy: Quality improvement measures with expert consensus. Health Literacy Research and Practice. 2019;**3**(2):e127-e146. DOI: 10.3928/24748307-20190503-01

[47] Lubash JS, Voiht-Barbarowicz M, Ernsmann N, Kowalski C, Brutt AL, Ansmann L. Organizational health literacy in a hospital-insights on the patients' perspective. International Journal of Environmental Research and Public Health. 2020;**18**:12646. DOI: 10.3390/ijerph182312646

[48] Ernstmann N, Hallbach S, Kowalski C, Pfaff H, Ansmann L. Measuring attributes of health literate health care organizations from the patients' perspective: Development and validation of a questionnaire to assess health literacy-sensitive communication (HL-COM). Zeitschrift für Evidenz, Fortbildung und Qualität im Gesundheitswesen. 2017;**121**:58-63. DOI: 10.1016/j.zefq.2016.12.008

[49] Palumbo R. Leveraging organizational health literacy to enhance health promotion and risk prevention: A narrative and interpretive literature review. The Yale Journal of Biology and Medicine. 2021;**94**(1):115-128

[50] Sentell T, Foss-Durant A, Patil U, Taira D, Paasche-Orlow MK. Organizational health literacy: Opportunities for patient-Centered Care in the Wake of COVID-19. Quality Management in Health Care. 2021;**30**(1):49-60. DOI: 10.1097/QMH.0000000000000279

[51] Kripalani S, Wallston K, Cavanaugh K, Osborn CY, Mulvaney S, McDougald S. Measures to Assess a Health-Literate Organization. Washington: Vanderbilt Center for Effective Health Communication; 2014

[52] Charoghchian Khorasani E, Tavakoly Sany SB, Tehrani H, Doosti H, Peyman N. Review of organizational health literacy practice at health care Centers: Outcomes, barriers and facilitators. International Journal of Environmental Research and Public Health. 2020;**17**(20):7544. DOI: 10.3390/ijerph17207544

[53] Briglia E, Perlman M, Weissman MA. Integrating health literacy into organizational structure. Physician Leadership Journal. 2015;**2**(2):66-69

Chapter 2

Literacy and Trust as Influencing Factors of Health Communication Online

Heinz Bonfadelli

Abstract

This qualitative research synthesis of empirical studies, integrated by a theoretical perspective, focuses on the societal and personal factors influencing digital health communication by individuals. In a process-oriented perspective, it analyzes how Internet users interact with online health information by seeking, receiving, interpreting, and using online health content with varying complexity, utility value, and credibility. The reception process, based on user parameters such as information needs, perceived benefits and costs, digital literacy, and trust, is influencing in a second-step health-related knowledge, attitudes, and behavioral intentions of Internet users and stimulates overt health-oriented behavior.

Keywords: health communication, eHealth, health information seeking, literacy, trust

1. Introduction

This qualitative research synthesis of empirical studies is integrated by a theoretical perspective and focusing on the underlying societal and personal factors that influence digital health communication activities by individuals such as health-related needs, perceived benefits and costs, and user experience on the hand and especially digital literacy or skills together with trust in online health offerings on the other hand.

The *digitalization of society* has transformed our lives fundamentally in all domains such as politics, economy, culture, and especially health communication [1–4]. Today, 96 percent of the population are *using the Internet* in the United States of America [5] and many say they are almost constantly online [6], and in most countries of Europe, for example, 76% in Germany or even 95% in Switzerland, and 86% also use mobile Internet [7]. In addition, more than 70% use the Internet and Social Media as *sources for news*, for example, 84% in Sweden, 82% in Switzerland, 74% in the United Kingdom, 72% in the U.S., or 66% in Germany [5]. Today, the digital media have especially for younger people become the most important source of information. And for the majority of people, the Internet has as well become the most important *source for health information* [8–13], for example, one in two EU citizens look for health information online, most popular in Finland and the Netherlands with about 75% [14].

This can be illustrated actually by the global health pandemic Coronavirus [5]: The coronavirus crisis increased news consumption substantially, especially for mainstream media like television, in all six countries with surveys before and after the pandemic had taken effect. And interestingly, trust in media's coverage of COVID-19 in 2020 was relatively high in all countries with 59%. And even 60% agreed that "media has helped me understand the crisis." [15].

But despite this society wide diffusion of the Internet and Social Media, there still exist gaps in access and especially disparities in usage of the Internet as the so-called *digital divides* in general [16–19] and especially for online health information seeking and application [8, 20–22], not at least based on varying digital skills to use the Internet [23, 24], especially among older adults [25–28]. In addition, there is the question, under what conditions health communication may eliminate health disparities [29, 30], especially in developing countries where still only about 45% have access to the Internet [21–31].

Not so long ago, experts from medicine and public health administration, together with the traditional mass media, possessed a *monopoly as trustworthy top-down sources* for health information. But this was weakened by the fast diffusion of the Internet since the mid-nineties under the label of *eHealth* and in particular by the new interactive Social Media with its participative Blogs or Apps as *mHealth* [32–35]or serious games with health topics [36]. Despite the benefits of those new interactive opportunities for horizontal health communication, there are disadvantages and challenges such as *social usage divides* [21] and risks for the users as well, because the search processes, for example, by Google or on YouTube, are guided by *hidden algorithms*, [37, 38] favoring in most cases the economic interests of the manufacturers of health or medicine products, for example, by *endangering privacy*. But even in the traditional trustworthy print media such as newspapers or magazines, there is more and more of the so-called *sponsored content* by health industry stakeholders in a similar form like the editorial content by media journalists.

2. A theoretical perspective of digital health communication

Figure 1 displays a systematic theoretical framework to analyze the complex field of digital health communication and to locate the many empirical research studies, dealing with a wide variety of online health phenomena [39]. It starts process-oriented from left side with the existing supply of online health information for different target groups, the usage, personal motivation, trust, perceived benefits and costs, and varying experience with health communication and its effects on health-related knowledge, attitudes, and behavior. This *input-output process* is embedded in a *macro societal context*, consisting of the providers of online health information on the one hand and the digital infrastructure on the other hand, depending on *communicative support* [40] by interpersonal communication of social networks [41] and the available resources by communities [42–45]. And individual characteristics of people such as age, sex, education, or a migrant background, together with individual information needs concerning health, perceived norms, for example, with regard to Corona vaccination, e-health literacy, and self-efficacy, for example, to handle Corona infection, influence on the *micro level* the digital health communication process.

Online Health Information as input can be differentiated according to its form and content. Of importance for the user are especially aspects such as accessibility and security [46], the visual structure of a Web site [47], the ease of use and user friendliness, and the complexity of online health information [48], together with its utility

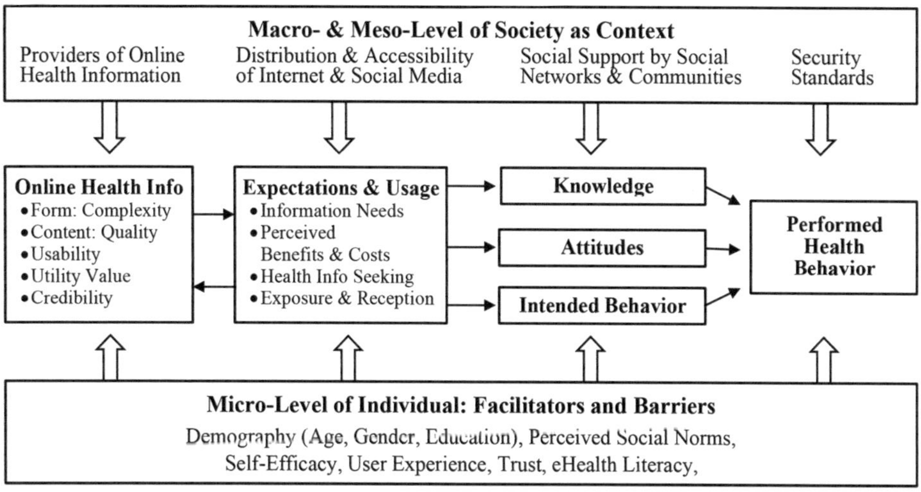

Figure 1.
Digital health communication: societal context, personal situation, use, and effects.

value, and not at least the quality and credibility of online health information and its underlying sources. There are many content analyses dealing with health information in general or with topics such as HIV/AIDS, cigarette smoking, cancer, body images, in the classic print media or television [49–50], but there are still not so many comparative analyses of *health Web sites* with varying interactivity and quality on the one hand and health videos in Social Media on the other hand [51–53] as a prerequisite for developing *Web site quality standards* [53–56].

Usage and Experience incorporate the many aspects of a wide variety of concrete interactions between online health offerings and its users, starting with *information needs, perceived benefits and costs* [57] and the process of seeking online health information and its exposure to it [8, 58]. And there are many *underlying mediating factors* such as *self-efficacy* [59–61] *online user experience* [62], *trust,* based on perceived quality and credibility of online health Web sites and its content [63–66], and not at least *eHealth literacy* [67–76].

Knowledge, Attitudes, and Intended Behavior of people are the effects of the varying use and reception of online health information, depending not at least on health information needs as motivation, perceived benefits and costs, eHealth literacy, and self-efficacy or trust, and are a prerequisite of the actually performed health behavior. Usually, there exist gaps between knowledge, attitude, and performed behavior, because of existing barriers such as costs or not having enough incentives or self-efficacy and empowerment [60, 61].

The above-mentioned interaction between online health content on the one hand and seeking and usage of this information by people and its effects on health behavior of users are influenced on the *macro- and meso-level* by the societal context, for example, with the amount and distribution of Internet access, the diversity of online health providers, and the social networks together with the urban or rural context of its users. On the *micro-level of the individual person*, there are mediating factors as well such as age, gender, education, or a migrant background that influence the existing health information needs, perceived norms, health literacy, and especially the *self-efficacy of a person* to seek, use, and implement online health information.

It is the aim of this contribution, to *summarize and integrate the existing research* and its manifold insights, focusing first on the processes of health information seeking, and second on the underlying and mediating factors of online health information such as user experience, involved credibility and trust, and health literacy, as well as the individual characteristics of the more or less active user of health online.

3. Methodology

The following summarized findings about the topic of health communication online and its influencing factors such as literacy and trust are based on a qualitative research synthesis of empirical studies from different countries and covering about the last twenty years. The considered results have been included on the one hand due to published relevant original research studies and on the other hand by citations in summarizing thematic publications, both have been searched in important journals of the field like "Journal of Health Communication" or "Journal of Public Health" and in relevant handbooks like "The Routledge Handbook of Health Communication," with a focus on publications in English language. Thus, the subsequent presented findings and insights of this review chapter are not based on a standardized quantitative meta-analysis, but as a limitation is only the result of a qualitative integrative synopsis of the topic by the author.

4. Health information online

Today, an immense number of *online offerings for health promotion* exist in a variety of forms such as Internet Web sites and videos on Social Media such as YouTube, Facebook, or Twitter, and with different levels of quality. And it seems that health Web site quality influences the intention to use it [77]. In addition, people use more and more the so-called *mobile wearables* such as Smartphone Apps that count undertaken steps or measure the cardioplegia, and give tips for healthy behavior like physical activity, but unfortunately often not based on clear evidence [10, 78]. Rossman and Karnowski [79] created a *classification, based on five dimensions*, that enables the contextualization of the wide variety of new *eHealth and mHealth Phenomena* (**Table 1**):

Provider	Addresses	Interests	Interactivity	Functionality
• Economy: For example, Health Insurances • Politics: Health Services • (Health) Sciences • Mass Media • Lay People	• Health Services • Politicians • (Health) Sciences • Lay People: General Public, Target Groups, Persons Concerned	• Non-Profit in the Public Interest • Commercial with Financial Interest	• Information: one-sided • Interaction: two-sided • Transaction: two-sided	• Content • Community • Provision

Source: Adapted from Rossmann & Karnowski 2015: 273 [79].

Table 1.
Classification of health offerings on the Internet.

There are on the one hand *providers* and on the other hand *addresses* of online health offerings, namely from governmental public health services or health insurances, from politics, (health) science and mass media, but as well from lay people, for example, as communicators and recipients, the so-called prosumers, of Social Media.

These providers of health offerings do not always represent *non-profit public interest*, but act as well as commercial agents with financial interests, for example, to sell medicines and drugs, however not always openly declared like in the many new health magazines. The online health contents can offer different *levels of interactivity* like one-sided information only, two-sided interactive communication, or even two-sided ways of transaction. And *functionality* means the purpose or the objective target of the online health offering like "*content*" as one-sided information for more or less passive receivers as distinguished from "*community*" as enabling two-sided interactivity between providers and addressees, and "*provision*" stands for supplying, for example, orientation in the doctor-patient relationship.

Not surprisingly, the *Usability of Health Information Websites* and *eHealth Offerings* [80–82]or the observed aesthetics [83] are judged differently by age groups: Whereas younger people prefer visually appealing and interactive content such as videos, games, or quizzes, and find too much text difficult to handle [57], older adults instead have difficulty in identifying and access relevant, reliable, and trustworthy sources of health information on the Web [27, 28]. In addition, sociodemographic factors like education influence the use of eHealth as well. It is a challenge that eHealth is still least used by persons who need it most [58]. To overcome these barriers, health information Web sites should not be generalized for all people, but suitably tailored to the needs of its specific target groups by taking into consideration barriers as well facilitators to enhance access, usage, and implementation [39, 84].

5. Online health information seeking

In most surveys, dealing with personal concerns, health has a high priority. As a consequence, it is not surprising that information seeking about health on the Internet and Social Media is performed by most people on a regular basis. **Table 2** lists data from different countries: In the Pew Internet Survey from 2013 [86], 59% of *U.S. adults* have looked online for health information in the past year, which means 73% of Internet users. And in 2013, 75% of the European population used the Internet and 59% of the Internet users were seeking online health information; the highest rates have been measured in Germany with 69% and Finland with 65%, and the rates increased in 2019 to 53% overall, but, for example, to 80% in Finland. There are as well survey data for Switzerland [85]: 92% used the Internet in 2019 and 76% of the Internet users have been searching for health information online.

Taken together, at least 90% in the Western Information Societies have access to the Internet today, and around 70% of the Internet users are seeking for health information. It should be kept in mind that most studies focus on *conscious and active searches for health information*, but not on "random contacts" with the topic, for example, on YouTube or Instagram. Furthermore, the effects of health information seeking on knowledge, opinion forming, and health behavior have so far been largely unexplained.

But despite the widespread use of online health information, there are still *barriers* such as costs and groups such as the elderly, the disabled or those living in rural areas, because of not having physical access, a lack of relevant digital skills or negative experiences with computer use [26, 29]. Ren et al. [87] analyzed the perceived benefits and costs of seeking and using online health information. Based on 282 questionnaires, obtained from patients and their family members, they summarize the following key finding: perceived functional, learning, social and personal integrative benefits

Country	U.S. 2012	Europe 2013				Europe 2019				
		EU 27	Germany	UK	Finland	EU 27	Germany	UK	Finland	Switzerland
Study	Pew Internet 2013	Eurostat* 2013				Eurostat* 2019				Latzer et al. 2019 [85]
Internet users (%)	81	75	84	90	92	87	93	96	95	92
Indicators	Health info online in past year	Individuals using the Internet for seeking health information				Individuals using the Internet for seeking health information				Individuals seeking health/nutrition info online
All** (%)	59	44	58	45	60	53	66	67	76	70
Onliner*** (%)	73	59	69	50	65	61	71	70	80	76
Sample	18+ years n = 3'014	16–74 years samples per country between 3000 and 6000								14+ years n = 1'122

Eurostat: https://ec.europa.eu/eurostat/databrowser/view/tin00101/default/table?lang=en.
**Percentage of health information seeking for all people.*
***Only for people using the Internet.*

Table 2.
Health information seeking on the Internet by people and Internet users.

positively affect online health information seeking, whereas cognitive (search) costs influence information seeking negatively.

Besides active health information seeking, a German survey by Bertelsmann Foundation [88] asked for the *communication channels used*, and the *underlying motivation* to use the Internet for health-related questions: 88% of the 18 to 80 years old adults have been seeking information about health in the past year, and 46% of these used the Internet as information source; the classical sources were still more used: 62% used mass media, and 56% had interpersonal communication with doctors or nursing staff or 54% with family or colleges. The most named *motivation of health information seeking* with 73% was to be informed about health risks and diseases in general; 58% mentioned to look for tips about healthier behavior, and the own need for help in concrete situations of illness (52%) or to be able to give help to family members and friends concerning health problems (46%).

But there are *dysfunctional aspects* of seeking and using online health content as well, especially in Social Media are the rarely transparent underlying *algorithms* a problem, together with *health misinformation* [38, 89, 90], as the public debate about COVID-19 is showing. As a *practical consequence*, there are *essential challenges* for the providers of prevention marketing [91, 92] and public health campaigns [93–97].

The above presented findings on the active search for information on the Internet and their underlying motives in relation to perceived benefits and costs [11] will be deepened in a further step by the discussion of some relevant *mediating factors* [87, 98–100], which influence the *modality of handling health information on the Internet:* namely (1) *user experience* like eHealth literacy [101], (2) *salience* of information about the topic, (3) *beliefs* that the behavior is producing the expected outcome, (4) perceived *behavioral control*, (5) *subjective norms* as beliefs about whether significant others think the behavior should be undertaken, (6) perceived *credibility together with trust* of site information [64, 70], and (7) *characteristics of users*. These mediating factors are relevant for providers of online health information, the tailoring of their messages, and the specification of relevant target groups. But it has to be emphasized that most of the existing studies focus on the so-called top-down offerings such as Web sites and online health campaigns; studies on interactive communication on the Social Web have so far been rare [22, 102, 103].

6. User experience with eHealth content

User experience during online health information seeking and use has a decisive influence on the success of an online offer and on its impact on users. The term user experience includes all experiences when interacting with an (online) health offer, starting with *navigational needs* [104]. Usually, the *subjective impression of health content*, its *usability or user-friendliness*, and the *attractiveness or visual aesthetics* of online health contents [83] are examined in corresponding studies [82, 105].

The way in which user experience as a whole and its various components work with classic Web sites has meanwhile been researched quite well, especially in the German-speaking countries. Right at the beginning of a visit, for example, access to a Web site or an advertisement in a social media feed, visitors get an impression of the visual attractiveness in less than a second, and this perception remains mostly stable [106]. And a high *visual attractiveness* increases the likelihood that an offer will be used for a longer time [107, 108]. For the willingness to revisit or recommend a Web site, content evaluation plays a decisive role [109]: Beneficial users are willing to accept any hurdles in usability for particularly good and exclusive content. Finally, *usability* is crucial for visitors to find search information immediately—or whether their experience of use is clouded by confusion, slow page construction, or navigational hurdles. And Uwe Hambrock [110] in his summary for the Bertelsmann Stiftung used qualitative interviews to investigate health information-seeking behavior of men and women in their role as patients in Germany. The interaction between doctor, patient, and Internet repeatedly revealed challenges, for example, when doctors advise against visiting the Internet. A key finding of the study was that information that serves one's own motives is more familiar in the sense of consistency theory.

For online offers, all the above-mentioned factors such as clarity, informativeness and likeability of content, its visual attractiveness, usability, credibility, and rating are essential. However, the research is still rather undifferentiated. Meinald T. Thielsch and his colleges [106] have presented benchmarks based on user experiences with Web sites as the so-called *user experience measures*. With the freely available collection of validated scales as a "*Website Evaluation Toolbox*," the key aspects of Web site perception can be recorded reliably. However, the subject of the investigation was classic Web site formats. Appropriate tools for analyzing the quality of other online formats have so far been largely lacking.

7. Credibility and trust

Another relevant factor for the assessment of online health information is *credibility of the information from a user perspective*. The credibility of information, or trust in (print) media and public authorities, but also in experts from academia, linked to keywords "fake news" and "lies press," has not only in Germany [111] been controversially discussed recently. Politicians are therefore trying to use new tools such as the "*Network Search Law*" (Netzwerkdurchsuchungsgesetz) in Germany to be able to follow relevant penal content better, especially by Social Media.

Research about the credibility of information and trust in these and their sources has so far been a priority for political news in the online sector. For example, the Digital News Report by Reuters of 2020 [15] shows that 45% of respondents in Germany still trust most news, with the extent for "news I use" being as high as 59%; however, only 14% trust the news on Social Media. Further findings also show that people rate *online misinformation* more credibly when they see it frequently [112, 113]. In addition, users with above-average social media experience tend to rate online information more trustworthy [114]. And the attempt to limit the spread of misinformation through warnings can even increase its spread [115, 116]. Information is also considered to be more credible when arguments are made for different sides of a point of contention. However, this rule of thumb depends on the extent to which the ability to think flexibly is pronounced among the beneficials [65, 117].

In the *field of health communication*, the research situation on trust has so far been rather thin; most of the analyses are limited to overall measures of "Internet" and "trust" without differentiating the formats and concepts [63, 118]. In Germany, Sarah Fischer [119] empirically investigated the influence of the type of information source and scientific uncertainty on trust in health services on the Internet with two studies. And Yeolib Kim [64] found in a systematic literature review up to 2013 only 20 English language studies that used differentiated measures of trust in Web sites. And he classified the factors that determine trust into individual difference antecedents, Web site-related antecedents, and consumer-to-Web site interaction-related antecedents.

And among the *antecedents of trust*, socio-demographics such as age, gender, and perceived health status, information quality, design, and perceived reputation of a Web site have been analyzed most frequently, but without consistent results. Sbaffi und Rowley [66] analyzed 34 studies until 2015. And they also were not able to find uniform results. Besides the role of *information quality* as a factor for the credibility of web-based health information, *health literacy* [70, 75] seems to influence perceived trust as well.

8. Health literacy

"Literacy" is a rather broad theoretical concept from diverse disciplines that constitutes a *heterogeneous and complex research topic* [67, 69, 70, 73–75, 120, 121]. It includes *different subtypes* that are strongly interconnected [71]: 1) *traditional literacy* as ability to understand texts, 2) *health literacy* together with eHealth literacy as ability to understand and process health information in everyday life as well as in the Internet and social media, 3) *computer literacy* as ability to use computer hardware and software, 4) *science literacy* as ability to understand scientific research and results, 5) *media literacy* as ability to access, understand, and use media content and its quality, and 6) *information literacy* as ability to know, use, estimate and process information. And health literacy and online health literacy, labeled as eHealth literacy, are strongly interconnected, not at least because most people today access, receive, and process health information not only by interpersonal communication in the form of conversations or the classic journalistic media such as newspapers, radio, or television, but as well by the Internet and social media.

So it is not surprising, that *many definitions of eHealth literacy exist:* According to Gunther Eysenbach [32], "e-health is an emerging field in the intersection of medical informatics, public health and business, referring to health services and information delivered or enhanced through the Internet and related technologies. In a broader sense, the term characterizes not only a technical development, but also a state-of-mind, a way of thinking, an attitude, and a commitment for networked, global thinking, to improve health care locally, regionally, and worldwide by using information and communication technology." In contrast, Cameron D. Norman and Harvey A. Skinner [122] defined eHealth literacy in a more concise way as the "ability to seek, find, understand, and appraise health information from electronic sources and apply the knowledge gained to addressing or solving a health problem." Not surprising, *the concept of eHealth* got many definitions over time, and a systematic review by Hans Oh and his colleges [123] found 51 unique definitions according to different persons like health professionals, consumers of health services, or lay persons using the Internet. In addition, there have been many attempts *to operationalize and measure eHealth literacy* on the individual's level, for example, in the form of *literacy scales* like eHEALS by Cameron D. Norman and Harvey A. Sinner [122]. But there is critique that the empirical measurement of (health) literacy was and still is mostly not based on a theoretical background, and literacy together with eHealth literacy is mostly measured based on subjective ratings by individuals and not on an objective factual basis. In addition, there still is not the so-called *gold standard of measurement.* And another weakness is that medical professionals have been only weak included in the process of definition and measurement of ehealth literacy [71].

As a significant factor in the field of health communication, eHealth literacy has been investigated and still is in many *empirical studies*. But most studies are measuring the level of eHealth literacy hold by the citizens of a specific population or by subgroups of a population only in a descriptive way, and especially in survey studies only as subjective assessment. As an example, the Flash Eurobarometer 404 survey investigated *"European Citizens' Digital Health Literacy"* with the following key insights by the European Commission in 2014 [23]: 1) Around six out of 10 respondents and 75% of the Internet users (80% of the population) had searched online for health-related information within the last year, the highest in the 25–34 age group. 2) Over three quarters of all respondents agreed that the Internet was a good tool for improving their knowledge of health-related topics. 3) Nearly 9 out of 10 people who looked for health information online said they were satisfied with the information they found. 4) Eight out of 10 people thought that the health-related information they found online was useful and that it was easy to understand. 5) And even more than 9 out of 10 respondents agree that their research on the Internet helps them improve their knowledge of health-related topics. 6) Over 80% agreed that they know where to find reliable health-related information on the Internet, and even 90% agreed that they know how to use the health-related information they found on the Internet. 7) But still 40% did not think the information came from a trustworthy source and did not trust information from the Internet to make health-related decisions. These results indicate an overall high level of online health literacy but can also be interpreted as an uncritically overestimation by many persons.

Beyond that, there has been the question if *eHealth literacy as a significant independent factor* is influencing whether an online health content is perceived and evaluated as useful and credible [75], a layout as aesthetically satisfying, or a media source or sender is perceived as trustworthy or not [70]. And besides empirical research, in practice there have been many *interventions* in the form of programs to improve the eHealth literacy of potential user groups like older adults [124]. The underlying goal especially in media education at school is learning how to deal with media by enhancing media knowledge and media competency of the pupils in form of skills to judge media reality more critically and, for example, to detect Fake News [125, 126].

9. Personal context of online communication

Besides trust and eHealth literacy, there are additional factors influencing health online communication. *Demographics* of persons and target groups such as age, gender, or education on the one hand, and the *personal context of online use* on the other hand also have an impact on the accessibility of the users as well as the use and appraisal of online offerings. And the significance of each factor depends not least on the personal context of health online usage. *Older people* for instance may not have access to the Internet together with the necessary skills to use eHealth. Otherwise, many young people today are particularly well accessible *via* an entry in their Instagram feed, which is scrolled through around lunch. In order to be considered in this context—for example with information on the effects of alcohol—a health campaign, for example, must be able to attract formal attention and interest in terms of content and be able to be captured in a very short time as well: This is not least because in this context of use the *attention span* is narrow and *cognitive processing* is rather superficial. On the other hand, young people are informed about a particular topic, for example, about the effects of alcohol on the occasion of a lecture at school, and seriousness, comprehensibility, and scope of information come to the fore. In this context, the *ELM-Elaboration-Likelhood Model* [127, 128] is distinguishing two contrasting "routes of information processing": A *central and in-depth processing* deals discursively with the arguments of a message, while a *peripheral and superficial processing* is oriented toward images and emotions. The consideration of such and other factors as well as the corresponding theoretical perspectives allows a more efficient approach of the respective target groups. A comprehensive model for online communication in the health sector would have to systematically integrate these conditional mediating factors and processes for seeking, accessing, and handling health information on the Internet as precondition of health behavior.

Valuable and useful information about mediating personal factors of health information-seeking behavior can be found in various models and theoretical perspectives of *social psychology* such as the *Theory of Planned Behavior* [129, 130] or the Social Capital Concept [131], and in *communication science* the *ELM Model* [127] or in *health sciences* [132] the *Health Belief Model* [133, 134] or the *Protection Motivation Theory* [135, 136], which deal specifically with health-related factors such as the magnitude of threat of a health problem and the vulnerability of people, together with costs and barriers but as well the usefulness and motivation of health behavior based on personal self-efficacy and coping assessment of how to deal with health risks. Not least the so-called *Transtheoretical Model* [137] also is of relevance for addressing the respective target groups, which distinguishes *process-oriented six different stages of change* in the management of health problems in which a person is looking for health information on the Internet as precontemplation, contemplation, preparation, action, maintenance, and termination.

10. Summary and conclusions

This contribution—initiated by Salaschek & Bonfadelli in 2020 [138]—provides an application-oriented overview of the development of digital health communication in the face of the Internet and Social Media, with a focus on online search for health information and its reception and effects, influenced by factors such as credibility and trust of health offerings by media and medicine, together with eHealth literacy as necessary precondition. In the studies carried out for this purpose, the *user experience and skills* on the side of the Internet audience, and the *perceived quality and credibility* on the side of the offerings of online health information are emphasized.

This results in *practical challenges for providers of health information* on the Internet and Social Media, but also for the planning and implementation of *prevention marketing* [68] and *online health communication campaigns* [93–95, 139], in order to still reliably reach the target groups in the new and constantly changing digital environment with informative, interesting, and convincing tailored health information that is perceived as useful and trustworthy [140] and should not deepen existing social inequalities [8]. And last but not the least, *empirical evidence-based evaluations* for quality assurance [141–143] play an important role for online health services, but also (certified) *quality labels for websites* such as the quality label "Health On the Net" (HON) based on criteria such as expert knowledge, data protection, transparency, and balance [144].

In addition to the active reception and implementation of the existing knowledge in communication practice [145], and in view of the existing shortcomings, further basic research on factors such as user experience, trust, and credibility of target groups of new interactive digital formats is important, especially for interactive communication on Web 2.0 [146]. And for application-oriented, various questions play a role, for which there is still too little reliable knowledge: In which reception context which target group can best be addressed with which formats? Or: What is needed to achieve trust, acceptance, and implementation in different user segments? Such research questions should take up the existing diverse practical experience, examine, and systematize evidence-based, to be able to communicate online more effectively and efficiently on health issues in the future. This is relevant not least because individual target groups like young people can already be reached almost exclusively online. But despite the ubiquity of the Internet, successful health communication will have to continue to work in future on an *evidence-based basis* with a combination of online and offline channels and offerings.

Author details

Heinz Bonfadelli
Department of Communication and Media Research, University of Zurich, Switzerland

*Address all correspondence to: h.bonfadelli@ikmz.uzh.ch

References

[1] Benjamin C, Potts HWW. Digital transformation in government: Lessons for digital health? Digital Health. 2018;**3**:1-5

[2] Helbing D, editor. Towards Digital Enlightenment. Essays on the Dark and Light Sides of the Digital Revolution. Cham, Switzerland: Springer; 2019

[3] Musik C, Bogner A. Digitalization and Society. A Sociology of Technology Perspective on Current Trends in Data, Digital Security and the Internet. Wiesbaden: Springer Nature; 2019

[4] Van Veldhoven Z, Vanthienen J. Digital transformation as an interaction-driven perspective between business, society, and technology. Electronic Markets. 2021

[5] Reuters Institute. Digital News Report 2021. Oxford: University of Oxford; 2021

[6] Perrin A, Kumar M. About Three-in-Ten U.S. Adults Say They are 'Almost Constantly' Online. Washington: Pew Research Center; 2019

[7] Latzer M, Büchi M, Kappeler K, Festic N. Vertrauen und Sorgen bei der Internetnutzung in der Schweiz. In: Themenbericht aus dem World Internet Project – Switzerland 2021. Zürich: University of Zurich; 2021. p. 2021

[8] Bonfadelli H. Digital inequalities in health communication. In: Hargittai E, editor. Handbook of Digital Inequality. London: Elgar Publ; 2021. pp. 217-232

[9] Bujnowska-Fedak J, Waligóra J, Mastalerz-Migas A. The Internet as a Source of Health Information and Services. In: Pokorski M, editor. Advancements and Innovations in Health Sciences. Cham, Switzerland: Springer; 2019. pp. 1-10

[10] Bert F, Giacometti M, Gualano MR, Siliquini R. Smartphones and Health Promotion: A Review of the Evidence. Journal of Medical Systems. 2014;**38**:9995

[11] Johnson DJ, Case DO. Health Information Seeking. New York u. a.: P. Lang; 2012

[12] Lustria MLA, Smith SA, Hinnant CC. Exploring digital divides: An examination of eHealth technology use in health information seeking, communication and personal health information management in the USA. Health Information Journal. 2011;**17**(3):224-243

[13] Percheski C, Hargittai E. Health information-seeking in the digital age. Journal of American College Health. 2011;**59**(5):379-386

[14] Available from: https://ec.europa.eu/eurostat/

[15] Reuters Institute. Digital News Report 2020. Oxford: University of Oxford; 2020

[16] Büchi M, Just N, Latzer M. Modeling the second-level digital divide: A five-country study of social differences in Internet use. New Media & Society. 2015;**18**(11):1-20

[17] Gui M, Büchi M. From use to overuse: digital inequality in the age of communication abundance. Social Science Computer Review. 2021;**39**(1):3-19

[18] van Deursen A, van Dijk J. New media and digital divide. In: International Encyclopedia of the Social

& Behavioral Sciences. 2nd ed. Vol. 16. 2015. pp. 787-792

[19] van Doersen AJAM, Helsper EJ. The third-level digital divide. Who benefits most from being online. Communication and Information Technologies Annual. 2017;**10**:29-52

[20] Brodie M, Flourno RE, Altman DE, Blendon RJ, Benson JM, Rosenbaum MD. Health information, the internet, and the digital divide. Health Affairs. 2000;**19**(6):255-265

[21] Chib A, Helena M, van Velthoven MH, Car J. mHealth adoption in low-resource environments: A review of the use of mobile healthcare in developing countries. Journal of Health Communication. 2015;**20**:4-34

[22] Moorhead SA, Hazlett DE, Harrison L, Carroll JK, Irwin A, Hoving C. A new dimension of health care: Systematic review of the uses, benefits, and limitations of social media for health communication. Journal of Medical Internet Research. 2013;**15**(4):e85

[23] Commission E. Flash Eurobarometer 404: Europeans' Citizens Digital Health Literacy. Brussels: European Commission; 2014

[24] Scheerder A, van Deursen A, van Dijk J. Determinants of Internet skills, uses and outcomes. A systematic review of the second- and third-level digital divide. Telematics and Informatics. 2017;**34**:1607-1624

[25] Friemel TN. The digital divide has grown old: Determinants of a digital divide among seniors. New Media and Society. 2016;**18**(2):313-331

[26] Hargittai E, Dobransky K. Old dogs, new clicks: Digital inequality in skills and uses among older adults. Canadian Journal of Communication. 2017;**42**:195-212

[27] Ware P et al. Using eHealth technologies: interests, preferences, and concerns of older adults. Interactive Journal of Medical Research. 2017;**6**(1):e3

[28] Weber W, Reinhardt A, Rossmann C. Lifestyle segmentation to explain the online health information-seeking behavior of older adults: Representative telephone survey. Journal of Medical Internet Research. 2020;**22**(6):e15099

[29] Borg K, Boulet M, Smith L, Bragge P. Digital inclusion & health communication: A rapid review of literature. Health Communication. 2019;**34**(11):1320-1328

[30] Freimuth VS, Quinn SC. The contributions of health communication to eliminating health disparities. American Journal of Public Health. 2004;**94**(12):2053-2059

[31] Makri A. Bridging the digital divide in health care. The Lancet. 2019;**1**(Sept):e204-e205

[32] Eysenbach G. What is e-health? Journal of Medical Internet Research. 2001;**3**(2):e20

[33] Kreps GL, Neuhauser L. New directions in eHealth communication: Opportunities and challenges. Patient Education and Counseling. 2010;**78**:329-336

[34] Schiavo R. Digital marketing the rise of e-health: Current trends and topics on online health communications. Journal of Medical Marketing. 2008;**8**:9-18

[35] Sundar SS, Rice RF, Kim H-S, Sciamanna CN. Online Health Information. Conceptual Challenges and Theoretical Opportunities.

In: Thompson TL, Parrott R, Nussbaum JF, editors. The Routledge Handbook of Health Communication. New York / London: Routledge; 2011. pp. 181-202

[36] Sharifzadeh N, Kharrazi H, Nazari E, et al. Health education serious games targeting health care providers, patients, and public health users: Scoping review. JMIR Serious Games. 2020;**8**(1):e13459

[37] Puaschunder JM. Big Data, Algorithms and Health Data. 2019. Available at SSRN: https://ssrn.com/abstract=3474126 or 10.2139/ssrn.3474126

[38] Shin J, Valente T. Algorithms and health misinformation: A case study of vaccine books on amazon. Journal of Health Communication. 2020;**25**:394-401

[39] Schreiweis B et al. Barriers and facilitators to the implementation of eHealth services: Systematic literature analysis. Journal of Medical Internet Research. 2019;**21**(11):e14197

[40] Kreps GL. Online information and communication systems to enhance health outcomes through communication convergence. Human Communication Research. 2017;**43**:518-530

[41] Wright KB. Communication in health-related online social support groups/communities: A review of research on predictors of participation, applications of social support theory, and health outcomes. Review of Communication Research. 2016;**4**:65-87

[42] Goldsmith D, Albrecht TL. Social support, social networks, and health. In: Thompson TL, Parrott R, Nussbaum JF, editors. The Routledge Handbook of Health Communication. New York: Routledge; 2011. pp. 335-348

[43] Lefebvre RC, Bornkessel AS. Digital social networks and health. Circulation. 2013;**127**:1829-1836

[44] Valente TW. Social Networks and Health: Models, Methods, and Applications. New York: Oxford University Press; 2010

[45] Valente TW. Social networks and health communication. In: Thompson TL, Parrott R, Nussbaum JF, editors. The Routledge Handbook of Health Communication. New York: Routledge; 2011. pp. 519-531

[46] Alajarmeh N. Evaluating the Accessibility of Public Health Websites: An Exploratory Cross-Country Study. Wiesbaden: Universal Access in the Information Society; Springer; 2021

[47] Valizadeh-Haghi S, Moghaddasi H, Rabiei R, Asadi F. Health websites visual structure: the necessity of developing a comprehensive design guideline. Journal of Paramedical Sciences. 2017;**8**(4):53-59

[48] Ford EW, Huerta TR, Schilhavy RAM, Menachemi N. Effective US health system websites: Establishing benchmarks and standards for effective consumer engagement. Journal of Healthcare Management. 2012;**57**(1):47-65

[49] Kaiser Family Foundation. Health News Coverage in the U.S. Media. January – June 2009. California: Menlo Park; 2009

[50] Manganello J, Blake N. A study of quantitative content analysis of health messages in U.S. media from 1985 to 2005. Health Communication. 2010;**25**(5):387-396

[51] Kristiansen S, Bonfadelli H. E-Health: Gesundheit im Internet. In: Rossmann C, Hastall M, editors. Medien und

Gesundheitskommunikation. Befunde, Entwicklungen, Herausforderungen. Nomos: Baden-Baden; 2013. pp. 237-255

[52] Venkatasubramanian M. Applications of qualitative content analysis: Evaluating the reliability and quality of health information websites. Qualitative Research Reports in Communication. 2021;**22**(1):89-96

[53] Zhang Y, Sun Y, Xie B. Quality of health information for consumers on the web: A systematic review of indicators, criteria, tools, and evaluation results. Journal of the Association for Information Science and Technology. 2015;**66**(10):2071-2084

[54] Devine T, Broderick J, Harris LM, Wu H, Hilfiker SW. Making quality health websites a national public health priority: Toward quality standards. Journal of Medical Internet Research. 2016;**18**(8):e211

[55] Eysenbach G, Powell J, Kuss O, Sa ER. Empirical studies assessing the quality of health information for consumers on the world wide web. A Systematic Review. JAMA. 2002;**287**(20):2691-2715

[56] Tao D, LeRouge C, Smith KJ, De Leo G. Defining information quality into health websites: A conceptual framework of health website information quality for educated young adults. JMIR Human Factors. 2017;**4**(4):1-19

[57] Reen GK, Muirhead L, Langdon DW. Usability of health information websites designed for adolescents: Systematic review, neurodevelopmental model, and design brief. Journal of Medical Internet Research. 2019;**21**(4):e11584

[58] Reiners F, Sturm J, Bouw LJW, Wouters EJM. Sociodemographic factors influencing the use of ehealth in people with chronic diseases. International Journal of Environmental Research and Public Health. 2019;**16**:645

[59] Ajzen I. Perceived behavioral control, self-efficacy, locus of control, and the theory of planned behavior. Journal of Applied Social Psychology. 2002;**32**:665-683

[60] Kollmuss A, Agyeman J. Mind the gap: why do people act environmentally and what are the barriers to pro-environmental behavior? Environmental Education Research. 2002;**8**(2):239-260

[61] Sheeran P, Webb TL. The intention-behavior gap. Social and Personality Psychology Compass. 2016;**10**:503-518

[62] Vantriet J, Crutzen R, De Vries H. Investigating predictors of visiting, using, and revisiting an online health-communication program: A longitudinal study. Journal of Medical Internet Research. 2010;**12**(3):e37

[63] Hesse BW, Nelson E, Kreps GL, et al. Trust and sources of health information. Archives of Internal Medicine. 2005;**165**:2618-2624

[64] Kim Y. Trust in health information websites: A systematic literature review on the antecedents of trust. Health Informatics Journal. 2016;**22**:355-369

[65] Metzger MJ, Flanagin AJ. Psychological Approaches to Credibility Assessment Online. In: The Handbook of Psychology of Communication Technology. London: John Wiley & Sons, Inc.; 2015. pp. 445-466

[66] Sbaffi L, Rowley J. Trust and credibility in web-based health information: A review and agenda for future research. Journal of Medical Internet Research. 2017;**19**(6):e218

[67] Berkman N-D, Davis TC, McCormack L. Health literacy: What is it? Journal of Health Communication. 2010;**15**(S2):9-19

[68] Bodie GD, Dutta MJ. Understanding health literacy for strategic health marketing: eHealth literacy, health disparities, and the digital divide. Health Marketing Quarterly. 2008;**25**(1):175-203

[69] Cameron KA, Wolf MS, Bake DW. Integrating health literacy in health communication. In: Thompson TL, Parrott R, Nussbaum JF, editors. The Routledge Handbook of Health Communication. New York/ London: Routledge; 2011. pp. 306-319

[70] Chen X, Hay JL, Waters EA, Kiviniemi MT, Briddle C, Schofield E, et al. Health literacy and the use and trust in health information. Journal of Health Communication. 2018;**23**:724-734

[71] Griebel L, Enwald H, Gilstad H, Pohl A-L, Moreland J. eHealth literacy research—Quo vadis? Informatics for Health & Social Care. 2018;**4**(4):427-442

[72] Ishikawa H, Takeuchi T, Yano E. Measuring functional, communicative, and critical health literacy among diabetic patients. Diabetes Care. 2008;**31**(5):874-879

[73] Nutbeam D. The evolving concept of health literacy. Social Science & Medicine. 2008;**67**:2072-2078

[74] Nutbeam D, Lloyd JE. Understanding and responding to health literacy as a social determinant of health. Annual Review of Public Health. 2021;**42**(1):159-173

[75] Paige SR, Krieger JL, Stellefson ML. The influence of ehealth literacy on perceived trust in online health communication channels and sources. Journal of Health Communication. 2017;**22**:53-65

[76] Samerski S. Health literacy as a social practice: Social and empirical dimensions of knowledge on health and healthcare. Social Science & Medicine. 2019;**226**:1-8

[77] Boon-itt S. Quality of health websites and their influence on perceived usefulness, trust and intention to use: an analysis from Thailand. Journal of Innovation and Entrepreneurship. 2019;**8**(4):1-18

[78] Chib A, Lin SH. Theoretical advancements in mHealth: A systematic review of mobile apps. Journal of Health Communication. 2018;**23**:909-955

[79] Rossmann C, Karnowski V. eHealth und mHealth. In: Hurrelmann K, Baumann E, editors. Handbuch Gesundheitskommunikation. Bern: Huber; 2015. pp. 271-284

[80] Guenther K. Assessing website usability (website management). Online. 2003;**27**(2):65-68

[81] Hinchliffe A, Mummery WK. Applying usability testing techniques to improve a health promotion website. Health Promotion Journal of Australia. 2008;**19**:29-35

[82] Thüring M, Mahlke S. Usability, aesthetics and emotions in human-technology interaction. International Journal of Psychology. 2007;**42**(4):253-264

[83] Thielsch MT. Ästhetik von Websites. Wahrnehmung von Ästhetik und deren Beziehung zu Inhalt, Usability und Persönlichkeitsmerkmalen. Münster: MV Wissenschaft; 2008

[84] Hardiker NR, Grant MJ. Factors that influence public engagement with eHealth: A literature review.

International Journal of Medical Informatics. 2011;**80**:1-12

[85] Latzer M, Büchi M, Festic N. Vertrauen und Sorgen bei der Internetnutzung in der Schweiz 2019. Themenbericht aus dem World Internet Project – Switzerland 2019. Zürich: Universität Zürich;

[86] Fox S, Duggan M. Health Online 2013. 35% of U.S. adults have gone online to figure out a medical condition; of these, half followed up with a visit to a medical professional. Washington D.C.: Pew Internet & American Life Project; 2013

[87] Ren C, Deng Z, Hong Z, Zhang W. Health information in the digital age: an empirical study of the perceived benefits and costs of seeking and using health information from online sources. Health Information & Libraries Journal. 2019;**36**:153-167

[88] Marstedt G. Das Internet: Auch Ihr Ratgeber für Gesundheitsfragen? Bevölkerungsumfrage zur Suche von Gesundheitsinformationen im Internet und zur Reaktion der Ärzte. Bertelsmann Stiftung: Gütersloh; 2018

[89] Southwell BG et al. Misinformation as a misunderstood challenge to public health. American Journal of Preventive Medicine. 2019;**57**(2):282-285

[90] Wang Y, McKee M, TorbiCa A, Stukler D. Systematic literature review on the spread of health-related misinformation on social media. Social Science and Medicine. 2019;**240**:112552

[91] French J, Blair-Stevens C, McVey D, Merritt R, editors. Social Marketing and Public Health. Theory and Practice. Oxford: University Press; 2010

[92] Grier S, Bryant CA. Social marketing in public health. Annual Review of Public Health. 2005;**26**:319-339

[93] Bonfadelli H. Gesundheitskampagnen. In: Kohlmann C-W, Salewski C, Wirtz MA, editors. Psychologie in der Gesundheitsförderung. hogrefe: Bern; 2018. pp. 383-396

[94] Bonfadelli H, Friemel TN. Kommunikationskampagnen im Gesundheitsbereich. Grundlagen und Anwendungen. Köln: von Halem. 2020

[95] Rossmann C. Strategic health communication. Theory- and evidence-based campaign development. In: Holtzhausen D, Zerfass A, editors. The Routledge Handbook of Strategic Communication. New York/London: Routledge; 2015. pp. 409-423

[96] Swire-Thompson B, Lazer D. Public health and online misinformation: Challenges and recommendations. Annual Review of Public Health. 2019;**41**:433-451

[97] Wakefield MA, Loken B, Hornik RC. Use of mass media campaigns to change health behavior. Lancet. 2010;**376**:1261-1271

[98] Lee T, Lin J. The influence of offline and online intrinsic motivations on online health information seeking. Health Communication. 2020;**5**(9):1129-1136

[99] Marton C, Choo CW. A review of theoretical models of health information seeking on the web. Journal of Documentation. 2012;**68**(3):330-352

[100] Wang X, Shi J, Kong H. Online health information seeking: A review and meta-analysis. Health Communication. 2021;**6**(10):116-1175

[101] Tennant B et al. eHealth literacy and web 2.0 health information seeking behaviors among baby boomers and older adults. Journal of Medical Internet Research. 2015;**17**(3):e70

[102] Huo J, Desai R, Hong YR, Turner K, Mainous AG, Bian J. Use of social media in health communication: Findings from the health information national trends survey 2013, 2014, and 2017. Cancer Control. ;**2019**(26):1-10

[103] Whiting A, Williams D. Why people use social media: A uses and gratifications approach. Qualitative Market Research: An International Journal. 2013;**1**(4):362-369

[104] Lee K, Hoti K, Hughes DJ, Emmerton L. Google and the consumer: A qualitative study exploring the navigational needs and online health information-seeking behaviors of consumers with chronic health conditions. Journal of Medical Internet Research. 2014;**16**(12):e262

[105] Shin D-H, Lee S, Hwang Y. How do credibility and utility play in the user experience of health informatics servics? Computers in Human Behavior. 2017;**67**:292-302

[106] Thielsch MT, Thielsch C, Hirschfeld G. How informative is informative? benchmarks and optimal cut points for e-health websites. Proceedings of the Mensch und Computer 2019 Workshop. 2019 Available from: https://dl.gi.de/bitstream/handle/20.500.12116/25258/642.pdf?sequence=1

[107] Lindgaard G, Fernandes G, Dudek C, et al. Attention web designers: You have 50 milliseconds to make a good first impression! Behavior & Information Technology. 2006;**25**:115-126

[108] Lindgaard G et al. An exploration of relations between visual appeal, trustworthiness and perceived usability of homepages. ACM Transactions on Computer-Human Interaction. 2011;**18**(1):1-30

[109] Bloch PH, Brunel FF, Arnold TJ. Individual differences in the centrality of visual product aesthetics: Concept and measurement. Journal of Consumer Research. 2003;**29**:551-565

[110] Hambrock U. Die Suche nach Gesundheitsinformationen. Patientenperspektiven und Marktüberblick. Gütersloh: Bertelsmann Stiftung; 2018

[111] Quandt T, Frischlich L, Boberg S, Schatto-Eckroth T. Fake news. In: Vos TP, Hanusch F, editors. The International Encyclopedia of Journalism Studies. Chichester: John Wiley & Sons; 2019

[112] De Keersmaecker J, Roets A, Dhont K, et al. Need for closure and perceived threat as bases of right-wing authoritarianism: A longitudinal moderation approach. Social Cognition. 2017;**35**:433-449

[113] Pennycook G, Cannon TD, Rand DG. Prior exposure increases perceived accuracy of fake news. Journal of Experimental Psychology: General. 2018;**147**(12):1865-1880

[114] Hocevar KP, Flanagin AJ, Metzger MJ. Social media self-efficacy and information evaluation online. Computers in Human Behavior. 2014;**39**:254-262

[115] Flynn DJ, Nyhan B, Reifler J. The nature and origins of misperceptions: Understanding false and unsupported beliefs about politics. Political Psychology. 2017;**38**:127-150

[116] Nyhan B, Reifler J. When corrections fail: The persistence of political misperceptions. Political Behavior. 2010;**32**:303-330

[117] Metzger MJ, Flanagin AJ. Credibility and trust of information in online environments: The use of cognitive

heuristics. Journal of Pragmatics. 2013;**59**:210-220

[118] Clayman ML, Manganello JA, Viswanath K, Hesse BW, Arora NK. Providing health messages to hispanics/latinos: understanding the importance of language, trust in health information sources, and media use. Journal of Health Communication. 2010;**15**:252-263

[119] Fischer S. Vertrauen in Gesundheitsangebote im Internet. Einfluss von Informationsquellen und wissenschaftlichen Unsicherheiten auf die Rezeption von Online-Informationen. Baden-Baden: Nomos; 2016

[120] Chinn D. Critical health literacy: A review and critical analysis. Social Science & Medicine. 2011;**73**:60-67

[121] Liu C et al. What is the meaning of health literacy? A systematic review and qualitative synthesis. Family Medicine and Community Health. 2020;**8**:e000351

[122] Norman CD, Skinner HA. eHealth literacy: Essential skills for consumer health in a networked world. Journal of Medical Internet Research. 2006;**8**(2):e9

[123] Oh H, Rizo C, Enkin M, Jadad A, Powell J, Pagliari C. What is eHealth: A systematic review of published definitions. Journal of Medical Internet Research. 2005;**7**(1):e1

[124] Xie B. Effects of an eHealth literacy intervention for older adults. Journal of Medical Internet Research. 2011;**13**(4):e90

[125] Jeong S-H, Cho H, Hwang Y. Media literacy interventions: A meta-analytic review. Journal of Communication. 2012;**62**:454-472

[126] Opree SJ. Media literacy. In: Rössler P, editor. The International Encyclopedia of Media Effects. Chichester: John Wiley & Sons; 2017

[127] Petty RE, Cacioppo JT. The elaboration likelihood model of persuasion BT—Communication and persuasion: Central and peripheral routes to attitude change. In: Petty RE, Cacioppo JT, editors. Communication and Persuasion. Central and Peripheral Routes to Attitude Change. New York: Springer; 1986. pp. 1-24

[128] Petty RE, Brinol P, Priester JR. Mass media attitude change: Implications of the elaboration likelihood model of persuasion. In: Bryant J, Oliver MB, editors. Media Effects. New York: Routledge; 2009. pp. 141-180

[129] Ajzen I. The theory of planned behavior. Organizational behavior and Human Decision Processes. 1991;**50**:179-211

[130] Montaño DE, Kasprzyk D. Theory of reasoned action, theory of planned behavior, and the integrated behavioral model. In: Glanz K, Rimer BK, Viswanath K, editors. Health Behavior and Health Education. Theory, Research and Practice. San Francisco, CA: Jossey-Bass; 2008. pp. 67-96

[131] Putland C et al. Enabling pathways to health equity: developing a framework for implementing social capital in practice. MBC Public Health. 2013;**13**:517

[132] Michie S, Marques MM, Norris E, Johnston M. Theories and interventions in health behavior change. In: Revenson TA, Gurung RAR, editors. Handbook of Health Psychology. New York: Routledge; 2018. pp. 69-88

[133] Becker MH. The health belief model and personal health behavior. Health Education Monographs. 1974;**2**:324-508

[134] Champion VL, Sugg SC. The health belief model. In: Glanz K, Rimer BK, Viswanath K, editors. Health Behavior and Health Education. Theory, Research and Practice. San Francisco, CA: Jossey-Bass; 2015. pp. 45-65

[135] Rogers RW. The protection motivation theory of fear appeals and attitude change. Journal of Psychology. 1975;**91**:93-114

[136] Floyd DL, Prentice-Dunn S, Rogers RW. A meta-analysis of research on protection motivation theory. Journal of Applied Social Psychology. 2000;**30**(2):407-429

[137] Prochaska JO, Redding CA, Evers KE. The transtheoretical model and stages of change. In: Glanz K, Rimer BK, Viswanath K, editors. Health Behavior: Theory, Research and Practice. San Francisco, CA: Jossey-Bass; 2015. pp. 97-121

[138] Salaschek M, Bonfadelli H. Digitale Gesundheitskommunikation: Kontext und Einflussfaktoren. Bundesgesundheitsblatt. 2020;**63**(2):160-165

[139] Bonfadelli H. Theoretical approaches of health campaigns and practical applications to COVID-19 campaigns. Science Journal of Public Health. 2022;**10**(1):60-72

[140] Noar SM, Harrington NG. Tailored communication for health-related decision making and behavioral change. In: Diefenbach MA, Miller-Halegoua S, Bowen D, editors. Handbook of Health Decision Science. New York: Springer; 2016. pp. 251-263

[141] Simon A. Qualität und eHealth. In: Fischer F, Krämer A, editors. eHealth in Deutschland. Anforderungen und Potenziale innovativer Versorgungsstrukturen. Berlin/Heidelberg: Springer; 2016. pp. 125-154

[142] Thielsch MT, Blotenberg I, Jaron R. User evaluation of websites: From first impression to recommendation. Interacting with Computers. 2014;**26**:89-102

[143] Thielsch MT, Hirschfeld G. Facets of website content. Human-Computer Interaction. 2019;**34**:279-327

[144] Eichenberg C, Blokus G, Malberg D. Evidenzbasierte Patienteninformationen im Internet – Eine Studie zur Qualität von Websites zur Posttraumatischen Belastungsstörung. Zeitschrift für Psychiatrie, Psychologie und Psychotherapie. 2013;**61**(4):263-271

[145] Corcoran N. Working on Health Communication. Los Angeles: Sage; 2011

[146] Welch V et al. Interactive social media interventions for health behaviour change, health outcomes, and health equity in the adult population. Cochrane Database of Systematic Reviews. 2018;**2**:1-23

Section 2

Trends

Chapter 3

A "Futures Literacy" Framework for Understanding the Future of Mobile Health Development in Africa

Ismaila Ouedraogo, Roland Benedikter, Borlli Michel Jonas Some and Gayo Diallo

Abstract

Sub-Saharan Africa is known to feature some of the weakest healthcare systems in the world. The expanding field of mobile technology in healthcare over the past years, commonly known as mHealth, has been considered to have potential leverage for supporting and improving healthcare systems, especially in disadvantaged areas, if people are literate enough to autonomously use them. However, implementing new technologies in African healthcare systems has not always considered local realities. Many African countries are facing challenges to capitalize on these opportunities. For instance, the lack of planning, foresight, and anticipation may affect the resources available for the implementation of mHealth. This chapter argues that exploring future scenarios can be a key point to successfully designing and implementing Health Literacy Mobile technologies for a sustainable healthcare system in Africa. The UNESCO Futures Literacy (FL) approach can contribute as a valuable foresight tool to anticipate "the future" of mobile health in Africa. Being "future literate" empowers the imagination and enhances the ability of African peoples and countries to prepare and co-invent inclusive health technologies that contribute to achieving both the agenda 2063 of the African Union and the UNESCOs 2022-2029 strategy. Overall, FL could become a catalyst to make new technologies tools of "liberation technology" and "justice technology" for Africa.

Keywords: Africa, anticipation, digital health technology, decentralization, Futures Literacy, mHealth

1. Introduction

The weakness of healthcare systems is one of the urgent challenges for Africa in the twenty-first century. The challenge in its developing countries is access to health-care, which can be problematic due to many factors such as lack of transport, long travel distances, etc. Less than half of Africans today have access to well-being facilities in general, and numerous African nations spend less than 10% of their GDP on medical services [1]. Fortunately, mHealth Technology can be a huge asset to alleviate these handicaps. Over the past two decades, a variety of mobile-phone-based initiatives have emerged to address these challenges. In the Sub-Saharan Africa region, much attention has been given to the use of mobile health to improve (1) education and awareness, (2) remote assistance, (3) diagnosis and supportive treatment, (4) communication and training for healthcare professionals, (5) disease and epidemic monitoring, and (6) remote monitoring and data collection [2].

Despite the advantages that mobile technology offers in the healthcare sector, many obstacles and challenges still limit the transformation of these potentialities into realities. Policymakers who take key decisions on mHealth implementation are often not informed about the positive and negative impacts of mHealth at different levels, such as the individual (e.g., patient care) and the organizational (e.g., productivity of hospitals) [3]. Also, they are rarely made aware of potential obstacles to implementation procedures and realistic timelines. Given the financial implications and systemic ramifications of mHealth, it is essential that policymakers and healthcare organizations rigorously examine potential problems about future use [4]. To study these questions, future studies, which provide different scenarios, are often used to help decision-makers choose and design the most desirable future. In the same way, technology foresight is used to support the prioritization of science and technology for promising investments regarding the future; the coherence and efficiency of innovation systems; and to create a common vision for the future of technologies, opportunities, and strategies in a more integrative view [3]. Given that complexity, diversity, and uncertainty challenge the mobile health sector in Africa, the more it is expanding, creative ways to engage with the future and to bring about change are required for the sustainable and future-ready implementation of mHealth projects.

In recent years, UNESCO has developed an encompassing contemporary approach to work with futures, as well as with future expectations and particularly with future-relevant imaginaries in specific contexts on the ground – an approach that is called "Futures Literacy" (FL). FL is a foresight and anticipation approach dedicated to enabling the capacity of individuals and organizations to become more "future literate." The FL approach has been instrumental in co-creating the new UNESCO 2022–2029 Strategy [5], which presents a long-term double focus on Africa and gender equality. It also coincides with – and is part of – the UNESCO Strategy for Youth and Adult Literacy 2020–2025 [6]. Although its practical value, to our knowledge, few studies have explored the use of this new approach in the healthcare sector and the context of Africa in particular [7].

In this paper, we present a visionary process in which participatory approaches and tools from the fields of futures studies are integrated into a new way of practical building and transforming the present by working with different futures according to the FL approach. The ultimate aim is to build sustainable healthcare systems to achieve the UN goals of sustainable development by 2030 and to realize the African Union's Agenda 2063.

2. Objectives

This study is part of a wider research project, which intends to develop a mobile health implementation framework to improve health literacy in rural areas of Africa.

Despite the tremendous opportunities that offer mobile technologies, Sub-Saharan African countries in particular face many challenges to implement mobile phone technology solutions in rural areas [8]. This study aims at describing the futures literacy approach and to show how it can be used as a foresight framework for mhealth in Africa.

The sub-objectives of the study are:

1. To give a general description of the futures literacy approach

2. To describe the environment of mHealth technology and explore the ways the futures literacy approaches can be applied.

3. To highlight some recommendations for using futures literacy in the context of Africa.

3. Description of futures literacy approach

3.1 Theory of FL

The term literacy has long evolved. Beyond the simple meaning of literacy or lettering that some attribute to it [9], we must now recognize that the disruptive advent of new information technologies has profoundly modified the meaning that the word conveys. This is hardly surprising considering that writing technology has always sought to increase communication. It's not easy to pinpoint a subject that is undergoing constant change. After some attempted definitions in 2000 by Organization for Economic Co operation and Development (OECD) [10] and the Canadian Council on Learning in 2009 [11], which were essentially limited to the social aspects, in 2013, the OECD eventually included "numeracy" in the definition of literacy as the attitude and ability of individuals to use sociocultural tools including information and communication technologies to access, manage, integrate, and evaluate information, to build new knowledge, and to communicate with others to participate effectively in society [12].

In that perspective where the concept of literacy evolves with the advance in science and technology, what should we think of the languages that allow machines to communicate with each other or with other people, or even to intervene in the future? Given that literacy increasingly involves skill-based techniques linked to complex devices. It already seems that the definition is not quite complete. Knowledge also deserves reconsideration [13]. In light of the progress of computational intelligence in particular the ability already to decode and produce both oral language, as well as neuromorphic engineering, there is also a place to review the notion of knowledge [13]. By processing data, machines also synthesize knowledge, all relatively artificial in so far as it is distinct from human knowledge.

From the massification of data and their algorithmic or computational processing, we can see a clear trend from the standardization of information and processes to their personalization. And yet we are only at the stage of weak artificial intelligence, which nevertheless manages to read certain texts more efficiently than humans [14]. This artificial intelligence, which is based on a Gaussian analysis of big data, will inevitably evolve, because the need is too great, toward an intelligence that knows how to process small data or personal data, in particular thanks to microprocessors with artificial synapses, which are starting to appear. Thus, by pairing it with human intelligence, we quickly tend toward hybrid forms of intelligence [15]. If the notion of communicational functionality has long been associated with the sole ability to process semiotic conventions, it appears that it is evolving toward the material technicality of devices. It is no longer enough to know how to read and write; you still need to know how to interact with devices to access information. Beyond the many ethical questions raised by the interference of technologies in what constitutes the essence of the human being, it is important to consider how the phenomenon risks further transforming the forms of communication [13].

Confronted with all these constantly changing information technologies, R. Miller argues the importance of futures literacy, that is, the ability to anticipate change [16]. This anticipation comes in several modes, for example, the ability to see change coming to prepare for it, and more constructively, the ability to shape or guide this change. It is from this latter perspective that futures literacy intends to explore.

3.2 Bridging the digital gender divide through futures literacy approach in Africa

Many empirical studies clearly show that women in the developing world have significantly lower technology participation rates than men; a result of entrenched sociocultural attitudes about the role of women in society [17]. According to Curtis Kularski [18], "the digital divide is composed of a skill gap and a gap of physical access to Information Technology (IT) and the two gaps often contribute to each other in circular causation. Without access to technology, it is difficult to develop technical skills and it is redundant to have access to technology without first having the skill to utilise it."

The large majority of women (an estimated four out of five [19]) live in developing countries, and they often suffer even more gender-related discrimination than their counterparts in developed countries; they are more likely to be unemployed and have fewer employment and educational opportunities [20]. These women are trapped in traditional family roles and lack the basic digital literacy skills that could allow them to achieve more of their potential [21]. As such, although it is evident that a gender digital divide exists in developing countries, it is difficult to know exactly how many women are accessing the Internet due to the failure of existing research to distinguish between the opportunity of access and actual use of the Internet; sociocultural factors are not taken into account. According to Moolman, Primo, and Shackleton [22], the gender digital divide is one of the most significant inequalities amplified by the digital revolution. Of the few studies that have sought to address Internet use specifically, most have found that women in developing countries are significantly less likely to use the Internet than men. Women are estimated to constitute 25% or less of Internet users in Africa [17]. In Africa (where the gender digital divide is thought to be the widest), in 11 of the 13 countries, more men than women use the Internet [17]. Controlling for these three variables (literacy, actively working or studying and belonging to the top income group), the gender digital divide disappears in most African countries.

As such, without careful planning, ICTs will likely exacerbate differences between men and women as diffusion and use of ICTs and their benefits tend to follow existing contours of income and economic divides, with the poor being further marginalized or excluded [23]. In that perspective, Futures Literacy as a scenarios building tool could serve as an approach to stimulate discussions around the choices that decision-makers in Africa have to make in responding to forces and uncertainties that bridge the digital gender divide and create a more inclusive digital future.

3.3 UNESCO futures literacy initiatives

As a pioneer since 2012, UNESCO defines futures literacy as a capability or a skill that allows everyone to better understand the future's role in their perceptions of the present. The term Futures Literacy can be likened to the idea of reading and writing because it is a skill that everyone can and should learn [24].

3.3.1 Futures literacy laboratory

UNESCO proposes that individuals can turn out to be more gifted at "utilizing the future," and more "prospects educated," on account of two realities. One is that the future does not yet exist, it must be envisioned. Two is that people can envision. Subsequently, people can figure out how to envision the future for various reasons and in an unexpected way. Since 2012, UNESCO has mobilized the latest advances in human thought and created the creation of more than 80 futures literacy laboratories. Participants are from very diverse backgrounds such (as governments, international organizations, and large professional associations). UNESCO has also created a network of University Chairs in Futures Literacy, which is growing rapidly around the world. The impact of these laboratories is direct, immediate, and tangible: the participants improve their ability to "use the future," It enables participants to make informed decisions for the present and acquire knowledge on a specific subject through practical experimentation. Participants can imagine the future for different reasons, using different methods and in different contexts.

3.3.2 Practical phase of futures literacy

3.3.2.1 In the first phase of FLL: Awareness

The first level is about developing temporal and situational awareness meaning a greater appreciation that change happens over time and that particular constituency, products, or organizations can be situated in time according to their values and expectations [25]. Participants are divided into small teams (assigned before arrival) in a way that facilitates their state of mind for the exploration of the past, present, and future [26]. In this first step of the phase, discussions are focused on what the participant thinks the next coming years will look like. Then move to what the participants want the next years to look like. They share descriptive portraits of how they probably and preferably imagine futures, without thinking about how we might get there. The objective of this phase 1 is to give participants a chance to say how they think it is and what will be.

3.3.2.2 The second phase of FLL

In the second phase, participants play a game that promotes a way of imagining creatively the future. As they invent and tell these stories about the future, participants become more adept at identifying and modifying the assumptions they use to imagine the future that shapes what they see and do in the world. The test for the facilitator is to produce a sort of "sandbox" so members can "play" with the "Learning Intensive model Society" (LIS) model to portray future edges [7]. The objective of stage 2 is to furnish the members with a comprehension of how to "let go" of the prescient and regularizing dreams of things to come off stage I dependent on extrapolation. It is likewise to help members think about past extrapolation and become more

Futures literacy	Tasks	Technique(s)
Level 1 Awareness	Temporal awareness, shifting both values and expectations from tacit to explicit all of which builds the capacity of people, teams and leaders to respond and innovate.	A wide range of catalysts an Processes generate the discussion and sharing of stories that elicit people's views on what they war and expect in the future
Level 2 Discovery	Rigorous Imagining (R1) involves two distinct challenges imagination and rigor, the former in order to push the boundaries and the latter so that what is imagined is "scientific "a and intelligible.	Escaping from the probable and preferable to imagine the possible demands systematic creativity and creating systematically, on-discursive reflection and social science are essential ingredients.
Level 3 Choice	Strategic scenarios are aimed at questioning the assumptions used to make decisions in the present, not as targets to plan-by but to provide new insights into the potential of the current world as a way to embrace complexity, heterogeneity and the pertinence of spontaneous actions that put values into practice.	Strategic scenarios are constructed using the capacities and stories acquired in developing Levels 1 and FL, by combining values, expectations and possibilities into scenarios that follow the narrative rules (see Level 1 FL below) and the methods of "history of the future."

Table 1.
Futures literacy tasks and techniques [27].

mindful of arising elective frameworks and have the option to portray a depiction of what the future may be.

3.3.2.3 In the third and final phase of FLL

In the last part of the session, the team focus on the actions they wish to take to address the challenges. Driven by a more subtle understanding of how the imaginary future participates in today's decision-making, participants are better able to appreciate the opportunities and threats of a changing world in new and unexpected ways. Therefore, participants are in a better position to identify actions and make decisions that they believe can help realize humanity's aspirations for resilience, well-being, and peace. The objective of phase 3 is to connect the discussion and description of Session 2 of the next coming years to our current situation (**Table 1**).

In recent years, several Future literacy labs have emerged in Africa. An FL lab was organized on December 8, 2020, in Gabon. Participants were called to explore the future of cities, youth, and perspectives for "peaceful and sustainable cities by 2050" [28]. A series of Futures Literacy Labs were also organized in South Africa first From September 08, 2020, to September 09, 2020, on the Challenges of African Urban Visions "Using Futures Literacy to Reimagine Our Cities" [29]. And then from March 31, 2021 to April 01, 2021, the University of the Witwatersrand (South Africa) organized another lab on "The Capacity to Decolonize: Developing the Literacy of Futures in Africa" [30].

4. How futures literacy approach can be applied to mobile health projects?

4.1 Overview of e-health and mHealth in Africa

The term e-health has a very broad meaning since it refers to all digital aspects affecting near or far health (see **Figure 1**). This includes in particular different types of digital content related to health, also called digital health or telehealth. More

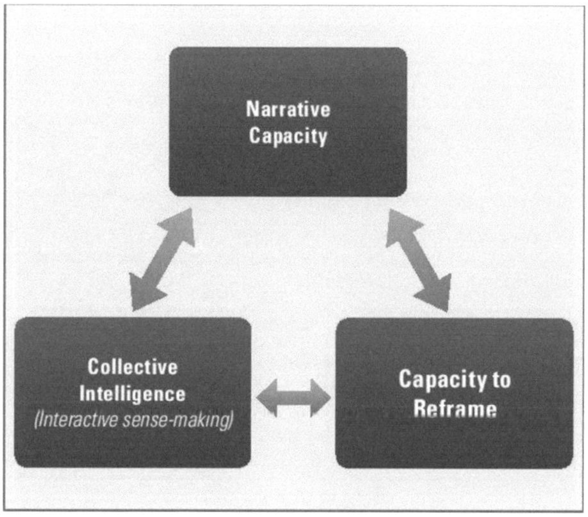

Figure 1.
Futures literacy as a learning process [27].

generally, e-health today encompasses innovations in the use of information and communication technologies in all activities related to health. E-health helps provide answers that will preserve the fundamentals of the healthcare system, while increasing its added value for professionals and patients.

Mobile Health known as "mHealth" refers to "medical and public health practices relying on mobile devices such as cell phones, tablets, patient monitoring systems, personal digital assistants and other wireless devices". African has shown great interest. Following the worldwide development of cellular telephony, mHealth technologies are seen to be a great opportunity, to improve the access to healthcare services in rural areas of Africa. The digital revolution in healthcare seems to be driven by the large diffusion and access to mobile phones. As indicated by the GSMA assessments Sub-Saharan Africa will stay the quickest developing area, with a CAGR of 4.6% and an extra 167 million supporters over the time frame to 2025 [31]. This will take the absolute supporter base to a little more than 600 million, addressing around a large portion of the populace [31].

Given the potentialities of mobile phones in training healthcare workers, prevention and health information, remote consultations, and patient monitoring are immense and are proving their worth in Africa. It is now a question of moving beyond the "pilots" to scale up projects seen to be effective and replicable. But for this dynamic to be sustainable and equitable, the use of Information and Communications Technology (ICT) for healthcare must be designed for and with caregivers and citizens, in other to respond to the priorities of national health policies and also be developed and financed with a long-term perspective with a sustainable economic model. (ICTs) project for healthcare and mHealth project, in particular, must be driven with a future perspective and strategic planning that involve a strong partnership with African governments and all stakeholders (**Figure 2**).

4.2 Applying a futures literacy approach to mobile health projects

As the National Digital Council of France underlined in 2015, as soon as the question of "health and digital" is raised, the subject becomes difficult to grasp as the expectations

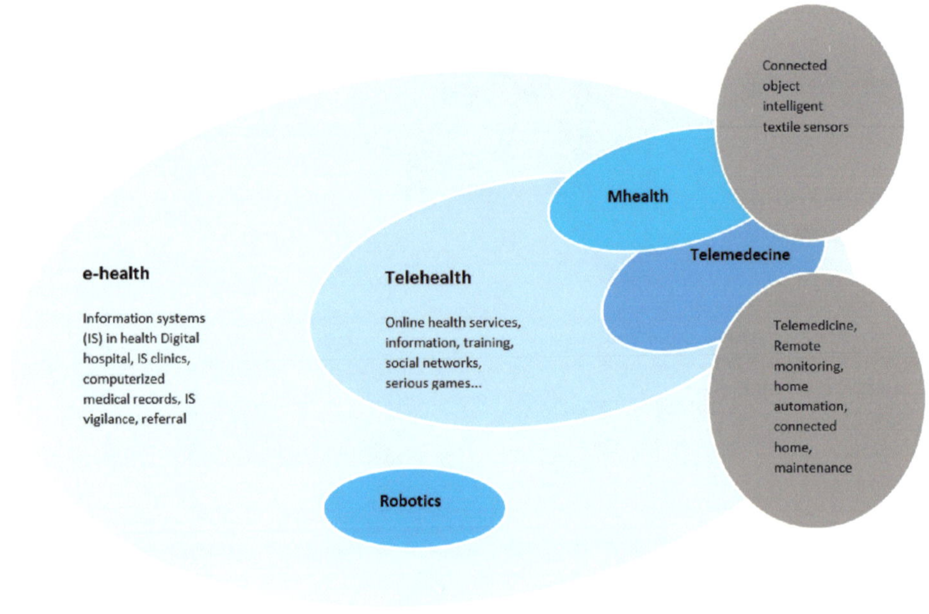

Figure 2.
E-health environnements [32].

and questions raised are numerous, complex, and often new. The profusion of innovations in the field of health that flood our daily news (whether technological, medical, social or of uses) and the variety of technological devices known as "e-health" even as we are in the context of care, make it difficult to know and take ownership of priority issues. E-health is presented by decision-makers or developers as one of the solutions to overcome the difficulties of our healthcare system. Promoting the quality and relevance of care and developing better coordination between actors are part of the ambitions of the reform of the health system and digital technology could participate. In addition, the specific issues related to artificial intelligence, which is increasingly used in several digital technologies in the health field, have been excluded from this note, as they raise new questions for healthcare professionals, but also for society as a whole.

In the context of "market" development, health authorities seek to maintain a balance between facilitating innovation and regulating it ethically. The so-called "e-health" field is very heterogeneous and refers to a multitude of technical devices, whose objectives and functions vary. Evidence of the effectiveness and service provided by these devices depend on many factors, including the pathologies concerned, but above all on the existence of evaluated experience feedback. The implications of the use of these devices for all players in healthcare and society as a whole are still far from clear. In such a complex environment, it is necessary to have strategic pacification tools to anticipate certain challenges and to achieve more successful projects. The futures literacy approach brings participants from diverse backgrounds to a workshop designed to make them think about the future in different scenarios. Using such an approach for projects, healthcare technology helps all stakeholders to get engaged with future perspective. Especially in a context where healthcare authorities are struggling to establish appropriate regulations for the use of mobile technologies and Artificial intelligence in healthcare, the Futures literacy approach can be an appropriate foresight tool to explore scenarios of the future for the integration of national healthcare systems.

4.3 Advantages of the futures literacy approach

The world is facing unprecedented uncertainty as the evolution of the COVID-19 pandemic weighs heavily on the economic outlook, leaders and decision-makers are forced to plan uncertainties and use Forward-Looking Technological analyses (FTAs) approaches. A future literacy approach was already undertaken to explore scenarios for future healthcare in Europe [5]. FL can help decision-makers react to likely directions in technology, manage risk, and shape technology trajectories to improve long-term benefits for healthcare systems in Africa. Analyses of emerging mHealth technologies in Africa and their implications are vital for healthcare systems and especially for rural communities. Today's global trends, uncertainties, and surprises have the potential to radically change the way the world operates tomorrow. This forced governments, businesses, organizations, and citizens to better understand the change and the future because we all live and work in a future world that promises to be different significantly today. Among the advantages of using the FL approach for mHealth projects, the following deserve special consideration [33]:

- It facilitates the ability to think and innovate new mHealth projects. FL makes it easier to take advantage of innovations
- It promotes detection and a sense of novelty, shock and surprise
- It disseminates a sense of initiative and experimentation within the community
- It simplifies (elaboration of various and varied possibilities)
- It helps to see truly differentiated strategic alternatives.

Due to the constantly changing technologies, Miller and Richard Sandford argue that scientific literacy and human is important to explore anticipatory assumptions [34]. This anticipation comes in several modes, for example, the ability to see change coming to prepare for it or, more constructively, the ability to shape our guide said change. It is from this last perspective that I propose to examine some forms that knowledge could take digitally assisted. Therefore, futures literacy can be a suitable approach to drive the implementation process of mHealth projects in Africa.

5. Policy implications and recommendations

To achieve aspiration 1 of the African Union Agenda 2063 "A prosperous Africa based on inclusive growth and sustainable development," each country must ensure that their citizens are healthy and well-nourished and that adequate levels of investment are made to expand access to quality healthcare services for all people [35]. Africans must also move beyond the trends of the past and go beyond the paths taken by other regions of the world. In that perspective, UNESCO and the OCP Foundation signed an agreement, in October 2017, to implement an innovative project entitled "Imaginer Les Avenirs de l'Afrique/Imagining Africa's Futures (IAF)" [36]. Futures Literacy (FL) as a foresight approach can significantly contribute to improving the ability of decision-makers to plan and use the future of African healthcare systems. As healthcare stakeholders acquire skills in LF which enable them to understand "the future" in different forms and perceptions of the present, they will "use these futures scenarios" to deploy "anticipation" strategies to respond to challenges related to healthcare projects. The creation of "future mHealth knowledge" through collective intelligence can be a good way to plan and implement mobile related health projects in Africa, especially within the framework of the UNESCO Global Futures Literacy Network. Opportunities must be given to healthcare stakeholders in Africa through FL labs to think collectively of hypotheses and future scenarios of new solutions of mobile health technologies to improve the accessibility of healthcare systems.

In the twenty-first century, new freedoms for development and advancement will be bounteously accessible in Africa. The landmass is as of now showing the world the path forward in regions like versatile cash applications. It is simpler to pay for a taxi in Nairobi than it is in New York. Stand proprietors in Zambia, not banks or telephone organizations, are spearheading new and safe methods of moving cash across the mainland, into the uttermost spans of the open country. The achievement of M-Pesa, and the broad accessibility of the portable stage, are bringing forth a large group of new businesses in Kenya. M-Pesa itself has ventured into Afghanistan, South Africa, India, Romania, and Albania. Many, if not the majority of these future chances were not accessible in the twentieth century. Quick urbanization, keen uses of mechanical advancement, expanded interest in the worldwide progression of individuals, exchange and cash, and also the constant drop out of environmental change, are molding new improvement real factors for an Emergent Africa. In the twenty-first century, advancement layouts from the nineteenth and twentieth century are quickly losing their importance. These "utilized prospects" address a world that presently does not exist. To understand the twin dreams of Africa 2063 and the 2030 Agenda, and to support the energy of arising Africa, we need to plan. This paper presents the utilization of vital premonition for better prospects in Africa to give nations experiences that will assist them with expecting conceivable future improvements of versatile innovation.

Foreknowledge is a key way in strategy making, as strategy making is regularly about getting ready for what's to come. The situation-based premonition approach, for example, future education can move expectant strategy making and backing the African readiness for future difficulties and openings identified with long haul patterns in the field of science and innovation as a rule and versatile innovation for wellbeing specifically.

The principal logical prescience pilot project helped the African government and the working gathering on Robotics and Artificial Intelligence to set up an administrative activity goal, received in the EP whole in Strasbourg on 16 February 2017, through which MEPs approached the European Commission to propose rules on mechanical and technology and computerized reasoning. Other than the foreknowledge-based approach, different thoughts motivated by the STOA concentrate on mechanical technology, fuel public discussion, for example, an expense on the additional estimation of robots as pay for conceivable occupation misfortunes, and the calls for moral rules for robot fashioners and clients.

Future proficiency can show us the potential chances and difficulties that might be the outcomes of continuous technological turns of events. It encourages us to feel more good with vulnerability, since we find out about the kinds of outcomes we need to plan for, and how we can pursue attractive fates and dodge unfortunate ones. This instruction clarifies how STOA utilizes the initially planned logical premonition approach practically speaking.

The primary key component of the methodology is picking points that may cause problematic cultural changes later on. We ensure that we have the most exact and exceptional data on the point. Investigation of potential effects follows—in an encouraging conceptualizing climate from different viewpoints, including specialists from numerous orders, particularly friendly researchers, to examine the cutting edge and potential contacts with specialized specialists, and applicable partners. Various viewpoints are ensured by "Soaks" (Social, Technological, Economic, Environmental, Political, Ethical, and Demographic), a plan that is utilized as an agenda to give seven distinct focal points to a theme, to guarantee that all potential results are investigated. The results of the encouraging meetings to generate new ideas are normally extensive arrangements of expectations and fears, likely proposed and unintended effects of conceivable future advancements of these technological patterns, including delicate effects (those effects that are difficult to quantify—for instance, influencing well-being, climate and security—and for which it is difficult to allot obligation). The distinguished potential results of future innovation improvements are joined in a bunch of different envisioned situations, built with the assistance of expert situation designers. At long last, investigating these envisioned conceivable future situations brings about top-notch chances and difficulties. It is these changes and difficulties that give direction to the African government in expecting conceivable future advancements through the work they do today.

6. Establishing a UNESCO UNITWIN network on digital health and AI for health literacy/education

We recommend an establishment of a UNESCO UNITWIN Network on digital health and AI for Health education. A network of universities in the North (University of Bordeaux, France, EURAC Research, Italy) and Universities in Africa (Nazi Boni University Burkina Faso). These institutions already have strong collaboration through many projects. Given the strategic position of these Nazi Boni University can be a coordinating institution in the South. The university is located in Bobo Dioulasso, the headquarters of the West African regional healthcare institution (West African Health Organization). Establishing AN UNITWIN NETWORK in this university can be an opportunity to strengthen regional collaboration between all the 16 economic communities of West African States. We recommend the establishment of a UNESCO UNITWIN Network on digital health and AI for Health education. A network of universities and research institutions in the North (University of Bordeaux, France, EURAC Research, Italy) and Universities in Africa (Nazi Boni University Burkina Faso) exists already. It will contribute to providing visibility and recognition to the work done by research teams in Africa and Europe in health literacy area. Health and education are both key elements of sustainable development. Within the network of 17 Sustainable Development Goals (SDGs), UNITWIN contributes to building and interpreting the evidence base of SDG 3 (Ensuring healthy living and improving the well-being of all ages for all ages) and SDG 4 (Ensuring inclusive education and quality for all and promoting lifelong learning). This UNITWIN initiative has a unique connection to UN agencies (including UNESCO and WHO) and is heavily focused on existing national networks. It is a source of strategic information production, knowledge transfer, and capacity building at both the national and the international levels. The UNITWIN network will be a "driving force" for networks, providing "think tank," "information-hub," and "bridge-building" skills that connect academics in Africa and Europe, global networks, institutions, relevant communities, unions, and local communities; operating at large and small levels of policy and practice. The network will contribute to the development of policy and practice through international research programs, translate research evidence, strengthen capacity building and provide support to policymakers and healthcare practitioners in Africa. It will also contribute to how the knowledge can be used efficiently and effectively in the health education sector. Finally, the project focuses on AI at the national, and regional levels and will provide evidence and guidance based on AI research methods, case use, deployment, testing, and exploitation.

In addition, the Network will be devoted to promoting the creation of Futures Literacy Labs on healthcare in Africa. The Network will focus on assessing and assisting in situations that allow for the transformation of healthcare systems through new digital health systems and supporting the development of foresight strategies and programs responsible for future health plans.

7. Conclusion

In this paper, we introduced futures literacy as a useful tool for strategic planning of mobile health technology in Africa. We argued that to achieve desirable results in mHealth technology, collective intelligence objectives and other criteria, a careful process must be designed. Futures Literacy as foresight practice brings participants, facilitators, and observers, as well as step-by-step process instructions for each phase together, including guidance on how to manage the dynamics of the foresight. Beyond increasing creativity, it also makes meetings more enjoyable and helps to energize the process of transformation concerning both the way an organization sees itself in the future and the way it conducts its daily activities by such a vision. Finally, some kind of participant debriefing or thank-you process should also be designed and implemented to inform participants of progress and/or to involve them more (e.g., an online network, newsletter, or discussion forum). This is important so that participants can be part of a growing internal and/or external network. Additionally, understanding the overall impact and barriers to implementation will help strategic planning processes be more precise. Successful implementation of mobile technology in the healthcare sector requires wisdom and the capacity to use knowledge, experience, common sense, and the foreknowledge of consequences, both positive and negative, of all the available courses of action to recommend the most advantageous option for the future. Sub-Saharan African countries have failed to prioritize health systems, something keenly felt during epidemics such as Ebola, and now COVID-19. One of the lessons Africa must learn from the COVID-19 pandemic is the need for strengthening its healthcare systems. More research is needed to explore each technology in more detail and assess its level of achievement over time. The project aims to establish closer ties with the existing UNESCO FL initiatives to build future technologies, which include artificial intelligence for access to healthcare for vulnerable communities in Sub-Saharan African countries.

Author details

Ismaila Ouedraogo[1,2]*, Roland Benedikter[3], Borlli Michel Jonas Some[2]
and Gayo Diallo[1]

1 Team ERIAS, BPH Health INSERM 1219, Univ. Bordeaux, Bordeaux, France

2 Ecole Supérieure d'Informatique, Université Nazi Boni, Bobo Dioulasso,
Burkina Faso

3 Center for Advanced Studies Eurac Research, Bozen/Bolzano, Italy

*Address all correspondence to: ismaila.ouedraogo@u-bordeaux.fr

References

[1] Clausen LB. Taking on the Challenges of Health Care in Africa. Stanford Graduate School of Business. 2015. Available from: https://www.gsb.stanford.edu/insights/taking-challenges-health-care-africa [consulté le: février 2, 2021]

[2] United Nations Foundation. mHealth for Development. 2009. Available from: http://www.globalproblems-globalsolutions-files.org/unf_website/assets/publications/technology/mhealth/mHealth_for_Development_full.pdf

[3] Hemmat M, Ayatollahi H, Maleki M, Saghafi F. Health information technology foresight for Iran: A Delphi study of experts' views to inform future policymaking. The HIM Journal. 2021;**50**(1-2):76-87. DOI: 10.1177/1833358319868445

[4] Wyatt JC, Sullivan F. eHealth and the future: Promise or peril? BMJ. 2005;**331**(7529):1391-1393

[5] UNESCO. Draft Medium-Term Strategy for 2022-2029 (41 C/4) and Draft Programme and Budget for 2022-2025 (41 C/5), Part I: Draft MediumTerm Strategy for 2022-2029 (41 C/4). France: UNESCO Bibliothèque Numérique; 2021. Available from: https://unesdoc.unesco.org/ark:/48223/pf0000375755_eng [consulté le: juin 2, 2021]

[6] UNESCO. UNESCO Strategy forYouth and Adult Literacy (2020-2025). Paris, France: UNESCO; 2020. Available from: https://en.unesco.org/themes/literacy/strategy [consulté le: Juin 2, 2021]

[7] Forte P et al. A futures literacyapplication in health care: The managedoutcomes project case study. Journalof Futures Studies, Taipei, Taiwan. 2020;**24**(3):51-61. DOI:10.6531/JFS.20200324(3).0004

[8] Muthiah G, Prashant S, Jhunjhunwala A. A review on challenges in implementing mobile phone-based data collection in developing countries. The Journal of Health Informatics in Developing Countries. 2011;**5**:366-374

[9] Souchier E. La lettrure à l'écran. Communication langages. 2012;**174**(4):85-108

[10] OECD. Literacy in the Information Age. 2000. Available from: http://www.oecd.org/education/skills-beyond-school/41529765.pdf

[11] Cathia B et al. Dans Littératie et numératie: Comment enseigner des habiletés liées à la littératie et à la numératie? 2014. Available from: https://www4.ac-nancy-metz.fr/ppem/IMG/pdf/ARTICLE_LITTERATIE_NUMERATIE_Version_definitive_2014.pdf

[12] OECD. Literacy, Numeracy and Problem-Solving in Technology-Rich Environments: Framework for the OECD Survey of Adult Skills. Paris: OECD Publishing; 2012. pp. 34. DOI: 10.1787/9789264128859-en

[13] Guité F. Le futur de la littératie. ACTES DU COLLOQUE CIRTA 2018: Présent et futur de l'enseignement et de l'apprentissage numérique, Canada. October 10-11, 2018. Available from: https://cirta2018.teluq.ca/teluqDownload.php?file=2019/03/13_Guite_Francois.pdf

[14] Pham S. Computers Are Getting Better than Humans at Reading. United States: CNN Money; 2018.

Available from: https://money.cnn.com/2018/01/15/technology/reading-robot-alibaba-microsoft-stanford/index.html [consulté le: mai 26, 2021]

[15] Kamar E. Directions in Hybrid Intelligence: Complementing AI Systems with Human Intelligence. 2016. Available from: https://www.microsoft.com/en-us/research/publication/directions-hybrid-intelligence-complementing-ai-systems-human-intelligence/ [consulté le: mai 26, 2021]

[16] Miller R. Transforming the Future: Anticipation in the 21st Century. England, UK: Routledge 15 B/W Press; 2018. 276 p. ISBN: 9780367855888. Available from: https://www. routledge.com/Transforming-the-Future-Anticipation-in-the-21st-Century/Miller/p/book/9780367855888 [consulté le: mai 27, 2021]

[17] Antonio A, Tuffley D. The gender digital divide in developing countries. Future Internet. 2014;**6**:673-687. DOI: 10.3390/fi6040673

[18] Kularski CM. The Digital Divide as a Continuation of Traditional Systems of Inequality. 2012. Available from: https://paper/The-Digital-Divide-as-a-Continuation-of-Traditional-Kularski/bc47c52d12fbe8dfbdaf6fb47488c74dca45ac63 [consulté le: juin 8, 2021]

[19] Hilbert M. Digital gender divide or technologically empowered women in developing countries? A typical case of lies, damned lies, and statistics. Women's Studies International Forum. 2011;**34**(6):479-489. DOI: 10.1016/j.wsif.2011.07.001

[20] Chadwick D, Wesson C, Fullwood C. Internet access by people with intellectual disabilities: Inequalities and opportunities. Future Internet. 2013;**5**(3):376-397. DOI:10.3390/ fi5030376

[21] ITU Telecentre. Global Digital Literacy Campaign for Women. 2011. Available from: https://www.itu.int/net/pressoffice/press_releases/2011/08.aspx [consulté le: Juin 8, 2021]

[22] Moolman J, Primo N, Shackleton S-J. Taking a byte of technology: Women andICTs. Agenda. 2007;**21**(71):4-14. DOI: 10.1080/10130950.2007.9674799

[23] Melhem S, Morrell C, Tandon N. Information Communication Technologies for women's Socioeconomic Empowerment. World Bank Working Paper; 2009. Available from: https://documents1.worldbank.org/curated/fr/812551468148179172/pdf/518310PUB0REPL101Official0Use0Only1.pdf [consulté le: Juin 8, 2021]

[24] Miller R. UNESCO Pioneers Futures Literacy. p. 4

[25] Miller R. Futures literacy: A hybrid strategic scenario method. Futures. 2007;**39**(4):341-362. ISSN: 0016-3287. DOI: 10.1016/j.futures.2006.12.001

[26] Miller R. From Trends to Futures Literacy: Reclaiming the Future. Victoria, Australia: Centre for Strategic Education; 2006. DOI: 10.13140/2.1.2214.4329

[27] Miller R. Futures Literacy - Embracing Complexity and Using the Future. Vol. 10. Singapore: Ethos Civil Service College. 2010. pp. 23-28

[28] UNESCO. 30 Jeunes Gabonais Formés à la Littératie des Futurs Reçoivent Leur Attestation. Paris, France: UNESCO; 2020. Available from: https://fr.unesco.org/news/30-jeunes-gabonais-formes-litteratie-futurs-recoivent-leur-attestation [consulté le: mai 26, 2021]

[29] UNESCO. Challenging African Urban Visions - Using Futures Literacy to Reimagine our Cities 0. 2021.

Available from: https://events.unesco.org/event/?id=1171322806&lang=1036 [consulté le: mai 26, 2021]

[30] UNESCO. The Capacity to Decolonise: Building Futures Literacy in Africa. 2021. Available from: https://events.unesco.org/event/?id=3893985247&lang=1036 [consulté le: mai 26, 2021]

[31] Groupe Speciale Mobile Association(GSMA). The Mobile Economy SubSaharan Africa 2019. SubSaharan Africa: GSMA; 2019. Available from: https://www.gsma.com/subsaharanafrica/resources/the-mobile-economy-sub-saharan-africa-2019 [consulté le: janvier 29, 2021]

[32] Conseil national de l'ordre des Le livre blanc du CNOM. De la e-santé à la santé connectée. 2015. Available from: http://affairesjuridiques.aphp.fr/textes/conseil-national-de-lordre-des-le-livre-blanc-du-cnom-de-la-e-sante-a-la-sante-connectee-janvier-2015/ [consulté le: janvier 29, 2021]

[33] UNESCO. Futures Literacy. Paris, France: UNESCO; 2019. Available from: https://en.unesco.org/futuresliteracy/about [consulté le: janvier 29, 2021]

[34] Miller R, Sandford R. Futures literacy: The capacity to diversify conscious human anticipation. In: Handbook of Anticipation. Springer; 2018. pp. 73-91. DOI: 10.1007/978-3-319-31737-3_77-1

[35] African Union. Promoting Health & Nutrition. Addis Ababa, Ethiopia: African Union; 2013. Available from: https://au.int/en/promoting-health-nutrition [consulté le: Janvier 28, 2021]

[36] UNESCO. Panel de Discussion D'experts sur le Projet de Recherche. Imaginer les Futurs Africains. Paris, France: UNESCO; 2018. Available from: https://fr.unesco.org/events/panel-discussion-experts-projet-recherche-imaginer-futurs-africains [consulté le: janvier 28, 2021]

Chapter 4

Important Role of Health Workers in Organ Donation at Gross Route Level

Mangesh Jabade

Abstract

Life is an energizing experience. It starts with birth and ends with death. Human spend various stages of life with different illnesses and issues between the birth and death. Donation of an organ is not the same as donating an organ or a portion of an organ for transplantation into another individual improving the quality of life of end-stage organ failure patients. The only choice is organ transplantation way to save lives. As a result, there is a supply-and-demand imbalance for donated organs, resulting in patient death. The number of organ transplants has steadily risen over for the past two decades, and children and adolescents have had outstanding results for their regain of life. That is why importance of organ donation needs to focus on gross route level in the community through health workers.

Keywords: health workers, organ donation, gross route level

1. Introduction

Life is an energizing experience. Which begins with arrival in the world and finish with demise. We spend different periods of life with various illnesses as well as issues between two of us. Healthcare advancement and technologies have started in order to protect people from death, and organ transplantation is most unbelievable feat in futuristic treatment, with the ability to save the lives of patients. Organ & tissue donation is integral to transplant. For post transplantation miracles is fully depended on polite judgment of donor & donor family [1].

An organ donation is not the same as donating any part of organ or organ would be inserted by operating procedure into another person. With case of end stage organ failure Strengthening patients' health and wellbeing. A only way to save lives is through organ transplantation. As a consequence, there is a supply and demand shortage for donated organs, resulting in patient deaths. Over time, REP Tree is a rapid decision tree method that automatically builds and prunes a judgment tree based on information acquisition, children and adolescents have achieved outstanding results. The increasing cases of transplant in elderly with comorbidity. On the other hand, is posing a problem. As a result of technological advancements and inventions in preoperative management, organ transplantation has improved [2].

Legally capable Persons can choose organ donation & donate body or entire body. Anatomic gifting of body by a person is individual decision for donation of organ. At the time of donation Family permission must be obtained. To ensure availability of blood & O_2 in organs until recovery of donor organs. This necessitates that a person dies as a consequence of An aneurysm, stroke, or car accident can result in a permanent neurological injury, which is normally caused by a major shock to the brain. The patient's name is checked against the state donor list to see if he or she has given their consent to donation in general. If a potential donor's name does not appear on the registry, the donation should be accepted by his or her legally authorized representative. Medical and social histories are collected as a donation decision is made. Organ donation experts Identify which Organs that are candidates for transplantation should be on the National Transplant Waiting List [3].

When compared to other Asian subgroups, Obesity and diabetes are more common among Asian Indians, placing them at a higher risk of needing an organ transplant. Coronary artery disease and hypertension may result from these conditions, which may Chronic kidney disease and other illnesses may result as a result of this. Dialysis is needed on a regular basis Organ transplantation can help patients with chronic kidney disease improve their quality of life. Diabetes and obesity, for example, may have a detrimental impact on an individual's life but contribute chronic liver disease can be led by fatty liver and, if left untreated, death, all other medications fail, necessitate a liver transplant [4].

It can be stated as universal problem of There is an organ shortage in Asia, but it is lagging behind the rest of the world. Also in Asia, India lags far behind other nations. It's not as if there aren't enough organs available for transplantation. Almost anyone who dies in a natural or accidental death is a potential donor. Even then, a large number of patients are unable to find a match. In middle of 20th century the development of organ transplantation has been a remarkable achievement. Awareness, support & active participation of people are needed for its success. It Without these considerations, the organ transplantation will be detrimental [5].

With a growing the number of patients in need Owing to increased Transplants, Many transplant programmes are attempting for larger numbers of surgical procedure from no cadavers because there are so many people dying on the waiting list and so few organs available. There are so many options for transplantation as living person organ donation is not only the choice. Have been hesitant to encourage it because it involves risky surgery on an otherwise healthy individual with significant morbidity and mortality risks. Given that dialysis is a treatment, choosing surgery on a healthy donor for patients nearing the end of their lives kidney disease it could be tough to explain, especially given the reduced quality of life of dialysis patients [6].

Preventing psychological damage, ensuring Donors are well aware of and want to donate without being pressured and tracking donor psychosocial outcomes are both psychological problems related to factors that have traditionally influenced donor behavior. Slowed the use of living donor organs. Inspiring the public, raising awareness, and keeping people accountable are all ways to overcome obstacles in the transplantation process.

Every year on 13th August Organ Donation Day is celebrated. Myths & fears in peoples is due to lack of awareness in relation to organ donation This day's purpose is to inspire ordinary people to pledge to give organs after death and raise awareness about the need of organ donation. To transplant after donor dies- hearts, livers, kidneys, intestines, lungs, and pancreas are among the organs transplanted into recipients can be termed as organ transplantation.

2. History of organ donation

Modern technology has given us a plethora of resources to aid in the donation of organs, but have you ever wondered where it all began? The following are some notable achievements and historical landmarks relating to transplantation of tissue and organs

- While some of the first known transplantation of bones attempts originate in the middle Ages. This field of medicine was still in its infancy. Without a doubt, those first patients and doctors were the best courageous people.

- While Bone transplantation dates back to the middle Ages, with some of the earliest recorded attempts dating back to the Middle Ages this field of medicine was still in its infancy. Those first patients and doctors were unquestionably brave individuals.

- It wasn't until significant advances in the field of science strong transplantation of organs became popular in the mid-twentieth century.

- Dr. Joseph E. Murray in Boston, Massachusetts, achieved a significant landmark In 1954, he performed the First successful renal transplantation (a gift from one twin to the next). In 1990, The Nobel Prize in Medicine was awarded to Dr. Murray.

- The first successful kidney transplants took place in the year 2000 on identical twins in 1959 as well as in 1960, and they were quickly followed by others by non-twin siblings in 1961.

- 1967 was a watershed moment in organ transplantation; it will be the first human-to-human communication, the first human-to-human heart transplant, as well as a transplantation of the liver, were conducted. Dr. Thomas Starzl, was a pioneer in the field of liver and kidney transplantation performed transplantation of liver. Christian Barnard, Ph.D. conducted the procedure, a well-known neurologist and cardiac surgeon in South Africa.

- In 1968, several significant events occurred, including the Southeast Organ Procurement Foundation was established after the first successful pancreas transplant (SEOPF), a specialist organ transplantation organization.

- In 1977 The SEOPF launched The United Network for Organ Sharing (UNOS) is a 501(c)(3) non-profit organization that pioneered computer-assisted organ matching. Programme of its kind (UNOS).

- The launch of Cyclosporine, an immunosuppressive drug intended to help In 1978, one of the most important breakthroughs in transplantation medicine was the discovery of a way to avoid organ rejection patients who have had a transplant Other drugs that are much more effective at neutralizing the rejection mechanism while maintaining the patient's health have since been established. Vital Immune system capabilities

- A human-to-human heart transplant, as well as transplantation of liver, were conducted. Dr. Thomas Starzl, a pioneer in kidney and liver transplantation, conducted the liver transplant.

- The first hybrid heart transplant was performed in 1981 under the guidance of Bruce Reitz, a prominent cardiothoracic surgeon.
- Dr. Joel Cooper performed the first successful single-lung transplant in 1983 and Joint Resolution of the Senate 78 established Nationwide Tissue and Organ Donors Awareness Week.
- The first double-lung transplant was conducted successfully by Dr. Joel Cooper in 1986.
- The United States alone, 200,000 tissue transplants were completed in 1989.
- In terms of setting criteria for organ procurement, a lot of progress was made in the mid-1990s. In 1998, France conducted the first complete hand transplant, followed by the United States in 1999.
- In 2001, In the United States, the number of living organ donors is increasing and reached a new record.
- The number of living donors outnumbered those who had died.
- A non-profit organization that coordinates the procurement and transplantation of organs (OPTN) established a website link in 2002 that delivers actual information on the total population of individual. In the United States, candidates are looking for transplantation of organs.
- In 2005, France successfully completed the first successful partial face transplantation, as well as Spain completed the first successful total face transplantation in 2010.
- Valencia's Hospital in La Fe, Spain, with Dr. Cavadas and his team, In 2011, a double leg transplant was performed firstly.
- 2012: The initial one robotic all parathyroid transplantation was conducted. Chicago's University of Illinois.
- 2013: The very first effective whole facial transplantation as an immediate life-saving operation was performed in the Gliwice, Poland, which has a section of the Maria Skodowska -Curie Institute of Oncology.
- The year 2014 marks the first time that a successful uterus transplant has resulted in a live birth (Sweden).
- In 2014, The first effective penis transplant was performed
- In 2014, the Transplantation of a neonatal organ for the first time was performed U.K. In 2014, the federal government's expanded definition of organs included law and rules included Vascularized Composite Allographs. (VCAs).
- Skin gun is invented in 2018, which uses a little bit of skin health that has been generated in a laboratory and Then it was sprayed on the burned skin In this manner, the Skin repairs in days, not months, and does not leave marks [7].

3. Criticality

3.1 Organ donation

It is a legal process where the organ of donor will be removed with his own consent or his near relative when he is alive/after death. Organ transplants is needed to comprehend. A transplant, is a surgical technique used in the setting of organ donation that restores function by replacing a damaged organ or tissue with that of a healthy person. It aids in order to improve the patient's standard of living and providing them with a second chance at life.

Transplantation will only take place if a donor organ is available. While the majority of organ transplants come Patients can also get organs from living donors in addition to deceased donors. People who are still alive donate their kidneys, liver, lungs, pancreas, intestines, or blood while living a normal life. However, the constitution states that the decision on deceased donors must be made by the deceased's next of kin.

3.2 Organ donation help with organ failure

It means second chance for organ recipients at a way of life Optimal health The heart, pancreas, liver, kidneys, and lungs are only a few of the vital organs that can be transplanted into people whose organs have failed. It helps to minimize the need for more expensive care following an organ transplant in order to survive. It assists beneficiaries in resuming their daily lives. A cornea or tissue transplant, for example, may mean the opportunity to see clearly again, or the return of mobility and pain relief.

3.3 Demand of organ transplantation

Organ transplantation is in high demand. India, like the rest of the globe, is experiencing serious organ shortages, with little hope of finding a solution. Renal failure affects 1.5 lakh people each year, yet only 3000 people receive transplants. Similarly, over 2 lakh people perish each year due to liver failure or cancer, and organ donors are in insufficient supply to help them. It's the same for heart sufferers: only 15 hearts are available for transplantation for every 50,000 people who have had a heart attack. As a result, widespread organ donation awareness programmes have been launched to close the supply–demand gap urgently needed in India. The statistics presented here are estimates; the actual figures may be much higher. This is alarming because it means that only a small number of people will be helped and given a second chance in life [8].

Ignorance and a lack of education are the primary causes of India's organ shortage. The benefits of organ donation are not understood by the general public. Today, social media and a variety of other platforms can be used to raise. The importance of raising social The importance of knowing the benefits of organ donors and also how increasing the amount of individuals who enroll for organ donation can help save even more lives. The organ shortage is caused by Misconceptions and myths. Most individuals are adamant about not donating organs. Due to the many misconceptions and superstitions that have been instilled in them, even after death. People with a pre-existing medical condition or the elderly are less likely to donate because they feel they are not qualified or eligible. If you have a serious medical condition, almost everyone will donate any or all of their organs.

3.4 Organ shortage is global problem

Not only in India, but all over the world. There are many reasons for shortage of organ such as knowledge about organ donation many studies which are carried out and many evidences are there which suggest that the people are having poor knowledge. The knowledge level is almost same for different category people such a people staying in urban area as well as rural area are having same knowledge. Students from regular degree and students taking education medical and dental colleges and nursing colleges also having almost the same knowledge regarding organ donation. The knowledge is same irrespective of gender, people working outside also and at home also.

Second reason for shortage of organ is myths regarding organ donation. There are myths that whole body should be intact even after death as to enter the heaven after the death. The religious person will not my last rituals if I do not have all organs. Body shapes changes after organ donation. Many believe that hospital removes the organ without their knowledge and consent and sell it. Many religious leaders are having misconception which they in thrust into their people mind telling about mysterious stories.

Third reason in availability of facility for organ retrieval and transportation facility very few centers working for organ transplantation and most of these centers are situated at metropolitan city. This make difficult for the people far from city to go for organ donation. Even if the complication develops, the nearby clinicians and physician does not take responsibility to take of such patients. That means they are least bothered for same [9].

To many legal formalities which are required to follow by donor as well as recipients. For this the donor may waste their workdays and wedges making them no interested to continue the procedure. Not only donor but medical fraternity also becomes least interested for the transplant procedure. The other reasons are there is no benefit for donor neither money nor any insurance coverage if they developed any problem in future. Government least interest, still government does not understand the importance of organ donation nor able to recognize the shortage of organ donation. So there are no measures have been initiated by them to overcome these problem. No specific policy or separate policies are formed only for organ donation so the procedure as well as donation becomes an easy or smooth procedure. The medication required for sustaining organ or to avoid rejection of organs many immunosuppressive drugs required which are costly so many times people find difficult to go for procedures as it is expensive. There should be measures taken from government to issues these medicine in subside rate. Awareness program and campaign are mostly carried out in the city level by NGOs which are comparatively vey less that is not enough to bring the changes among the people.

As people have poor knowledge does the attitude and practices towards organ donation. Many times people registered themselves for organ donation but does not make their near one aware about it. Which makes organ removal more difficult after death.

Scams of organ donation many people take disadvantage of this needy one and exploit the poor by selling and buying the organs. Making duplicate papers and creating problem for same. Awareness about the shortage of organ as people are not aware about organ donation so they even not aware that there is shortage and we should do something to overcome the problem. It even true with social media no media will take interest for doing propaganda of organ shortage unless any celebrity is involved in it. But they will be in front to advertise or giving news of scams by adding very nonspecific things in it. According to study there are few myths such as organ donation is not necessary in India, my religion discourages organ donation and organ removed will disfigure the body and affect cremation. Rejection of organ is also measure problem as people are worried about it. It requires special care while doing organ transplantation certain tests are carried out like tissue typing and matching, typing and matching of red blood cells and leucocyte cross matching etc. The number of tests also different according to individual requirement. Many times the test depend on the individuals defense mechanism some cell are active and fight and produce antigens against antibody very fast while some cells act as non-self-cells which will not require a tissue matching. It is also if we wanted to prevent rejection it is important that patients own relative especially those sharing a common genetic formation are come forward for organ donation. So along with this education of people and making them aware about it all thing is necessary.

According to Organ Retrieval Banking (ORBA) among many other country who is facing the organ shortage and India is one among them who is facing an acute shortage of organ. There are many reasons for this such as prevalence of myths and superstition regarding organ donation. The one more reason is poor knowledge regarding it. Many studies also found that not only rural but urban people also having poor knowledge about organ donation. There are also few studies which suggest even medical and nursing student has poor knowledge. Other reasons for shortage are unavailability of resources for donation and limited support for money incentives. The lack of knowledge and People's knowledge of sick organ donation is low, and many arc ignorant of brain death. How it is diagnosed how the organ from brain death person can be utilizing properly, practices like kidney rackets and exploitation of needy and poor procedure [10].

The problem is not only related to donors but also training regarding whole procedures. A study carried regarding this said that the physician's attitude towards the renal transplant patients and their follow up is very important. The study also specifies that during the treatment of such patients proper monitoring of the immune suppressive drugs level is important for that well equipped laboratories are needed as well as experts and proper protocol is needed which is not available.

According study carried out the regarding organ donation also suggested that those working in this team should have proper training regarding whole procedure which will help for its success.

Dr. Shingare, Director of DEMR Maharashtra in his opinion on kidney scam says that there should be campaign to spread awareness about organ donation.

Dr. Prashant Borahade on the day of organ donation said that convincing people for organ donation is a challenge, but if we are preparing people in advance the myths will be dispelled.

To increase organ pledges significantly state should adopt the law and guidelines and report data to make the registries more effective says Dr. Bhandari the director of NOTTO. Highlighting the need for capacity building and spreading awareness the aspects specified are all should worked on for a smooth and transparent donation mechanism.

Even now many feel pledging organs may deprive a donor of the best of treatment. A family may get harassed while claiming a near one's body. There are fear that organs may go waste due to an inefficient system and time lag. People want to know how organs are being used.

In India, 1.5 lakh people need kidney transplants, with just They will be distributed to 3000 people. Just one in every thirty people receives a kidney transplant, and

90% of those who wait die for a donor. Seventy percent of liver transplants need a live donor, while thirty percent require deceased donors. As a result, increasing organ donation rates is critical for giving people a second chance at life.

Comprehensive & scientific knowledge is needed for Organ and tissue transplant. They include assessing and managing Educating and counseling. If they are dead donors, transplantation receivers, donors who may be interested, or alive donors, they can take care of themselves, live a healthy life, and die happily when the time comes is close. For improving post-transplant & QOL this is important.

3.5 Legal position on organ donation

Organ donation is permitted under Indian law, man. The Indian Parliament passed the Transplant of Human Organs Act (THOA) in 1994, legalizing "death" and organ donation.

The gradual and permanent cessation of all brain functions is known as brain death. In cases of brain death, a person's essential body functions can be preserved in a 'intensive care unit' for a limited time.' Artificial help is provided to such people in order to keep their organs alive. Oxygenated and stable until they are removed. These patients' organs may be transplanted into terminally ill patients.

Health worker have a significant impact on the development of an effective transplantation programme They're vital members of the team that uses scientific, organizational, and human resources to treat patients and their families, with the aim of organizing, caring for, informing, and performing Donation of organs and tissues, as well as transplantation studies. As a result, health care professionals must be well-versed in ethical values and should have expertise at their disposal to identify patient complications and social problems relevant organ donation and transplantation Future research into the positions and duties of health staff is hoped for by the researchers.

4. Problem on hand

The kidney was the 1st human organ to be successfully transplanted in 1954. Long-term and intestinal organ transplants started in the 1980s, following active liver, heart, and pancreatic transplants at the end of 1906. Core, kidneys, brain, liver, lungs, pancreas, intestines, and thalamus transplants have all been successful. Among the tissues are the bone, tendons, skin, eyes, heart muscle, nerves, and veins are all examples of connective tissue. The kidneys, liver, brain, eye, and orthopedic tissue are the most frequently transplanted organs, followed by liver, heart, cornea, and musculoskeletal tissue [11].

Skin transplantation is dealt with in the early stages of transplantation. The first rational account Sushrata, an Indian surgeon who lived in the second century BEFORE CHRIST, gave this advice. In the nose reconstruction, he performed a rhino-plasty with autographed skin transplantation. The success or failure of these procedures is unknown. Surgeon Gaspro Tagliacozzi of Italy performed excellent skin auto-grafts centuries later, but he struggled with allografts on a regular basis, providing the first sign of rejection centuries before the method was fully understood. In 1954, at Brigham and Women's Hospital in Boston, the very first effective organ transplant was conducted which he credited to the "heart and strength of individual-ism." The procedure was carried out by For his work, Dr. Joseph Murray was given the Nobel Prize in Medicine [12].

Eduard Zirm (Olomouc eye clinic) performed the first cornea transplant in 1905, making it one of the first popular types of transplant surgery. The establishment of eye banks was crucial to the success of cornea transplantation. These are non-profit organizations that organize the distribution of donated corneas to surgeons and provide eyes for research around the world. In 1967, South Africa was the site of the world's The very first heart transplantation was performed In the year 1968, at Sydney's St Vincent's Hospital. The first successful lung transplantation operation was conducted in 1981 by Stanford University's Dr. Bruce Reitz on a patient with idiopathic pulmonary hypertension. Thomas Starzl conducted the first human liver transplant in 1963, but the pediatric patient died during the procedure as a result of uncontrollable bleeding after multiple attempts by various surgeons failed, a 19-month-old girl with hepatocellular cancer was transplanted by Starzl, who lived for more than a year before dying of metastatic cancer. Despite advances in surgical methods, liver transplantation was still considered experimental until the 1970s, with just a 25% one-year patient survival rate. Thanks to advances in medicine, liver transplantation became a popular clinical practice in the 1980s, Sir Roy Clane, Professor of Surgery at Cambridge, discovered cyclosporine and it was used to treat both adults and children with suitable grounds [13].

5. Need of the study

As per WHO principle 3- Donations from the deceased should be established so that their full therapeutic potential can be realized in order to reduce the risk to living donors. as much as possible. The effectiveness of deceased donation programmes is dependent on communities and health professionals being more knowledgeable about donation and transplantation.

Despite the extensive use of deceased donor materials, living donor donations are needed for some types of transplants or to compensate for the limited supply of deceased donor materials in order to meet patient needs. Despite the fact that living donation carries certain risks for the donor that aren't insignificant, it is nevertheless practiced.

Since finding Human tissue for transplantation from deceased or living donors, as well as allogeneic For both the recipient and the donor, Since transplantation can pose ethical and safety concerns, health officials should enforce strict controls and adequate monitoring to safeguard patients. The Guiding Principles require that donors and beneficiaries be treated as humanely as possible.

Over 500,000 people from India are expected to need organ transplantation in the United States.

- Due to organs aren't available 5 million people perish.
- Due to liver disease 2 lakhs people die
- With heart diseases 50,000 people die
- From 150,000 people only five thousand get kidney transplant
- Ten lakhs Individuals who are corneal blind and awaiting transplantation

Despite this, Per year, less than a thousand deceased donor transplants are performed, a tiny and negligible amount as compared to global statistics. Any of these patients may be eligible For organ transplantation A living donor. The others are almost certainly going to die while waiting for an organ transplant.

To comprehend understand Before you can donate an organ, you must first learn about transplanting of organs. A graft is a medical operation that involves the removal of a part of the body. That restores the function of a damaged organ or tissue from one person by replacing it with healthy tissue from another person. Despite major advances in medical science, transplantation remains the only alternative in some cases. Transplants increase a patient's quality of life and provide them with a new lease on life.

A transplant may Only if an organ from a donor is available can this procedure be carried out. Although the majority of organ transplants come from deceased donors, patients may also get organs from living donors. Living individuals will donate a kidney, a portion of their liver, lungs, pancreas, intestines, and blood while continuing to live normal lives. However, according to the constitution, the decision on deceased donors ultimately lies with the relatives of the dead.

Because of organ A transplant also means a second chance of life for recipients. The heart, the pancreas, the liver, the kidney and the lungs are only a few of the essential organs that can be transplanted into people who have failed to have their organs function properly. For certain people, receiving an organ transplant means no longer having to undergo expensive routine operations to stay alive. Many people are able to regain their daily lives as a result of it.

Past Thousands of people Since first successful organ transplantation 50 years ago, their lives have been extended and their health has improved in the United States as well as the rest of the world. Thanks to transplanted kidneys, hearts, pancreas, livers, and other strong organs.

The blood donation and transplant program's goal is to utilize all donated organs to prolong or enhance the lives for transplant recipients. As a consequence of advances in fundamental and clinical research over the past several decades, organ transplantation has become the sole treatment for a large number of end-stage organ-specific illnesses. However, there are insufficient organ donations to satisfy the need. Furthermore, some organs may not be recoverable, others may not be transplantable, and some organ transplants may fail, all of which add to the supply–demand imbalance. The health of the donor, the cause of death, and functional or anatomic abnormalities discovered in a prospective donor or donor organ are all factors that influence whether or not an organ is appropriate for transplantation. To date, most organ transplant research has concentrated on transplant recipients and ways to boost transplant and post-transplant health outcomes. It has taken a long time for improvements in the number and quality of organs eligible for transplantation to occur, with the majority of them owing to changes in local practice criteria. Researching deceased organ donors and organs obtained from deceased donors has emerged as one way to find novel approaches to increase the amount and quality of organs that can be successfully transplanted, thus increasing the number of patients who obtain a functional organ.

Many lives could be saved if organs from cadaver donors were available. Every year in India, thousands of people die as an outcome of the difficulty or inability of transplanting unpa/ired organs like the heart, liver, and pancreas from living donors.

Progresses Despite the fact that medical science has made critical human organ transplantation possible, millions of people in India are still losing their lives due to a scarcity of donors. Every year, In India, more than 1.5 million people have been identified with end-stage renal disease as a result of cancer. However, only a few thousand transplants are performed each year, and patients are forced to rely on dialysis to survive.

6. Organ donation statistics

6.1 Global

The database on donation and transplantation is the most extensive collection of worldwide data derived from official sources on organ donation & transplantation activities, as well as legal and organizational information. Organ transplanted annually (2016): 1, 35,860. It increases over 2015 by: 7.25% Actual deceased organ donors in 2016 are: 34,854,Transplants per hour in 2016 by:15.5% Living kidney transplants 2016 are – 40%, Actual DCD (deceased 2016 are – 19%, Living liver transplants 2016 are – 19%.

More than 36,500 transplants were performed in 2018, giving patients, their families, and their communities new leases on life (from more than 10,700 deceased and 6800 living donors).

- In 2020, the number of people who received transplants decreased by 13% compared to 2019, while the number of donors decreased by 16%.

- Around 1650 Australians are waiting for the purpose of a renal transplantation, There are more than 12,000 people on dialysis, even those in serious need of a transplant.

- Thanks to the kindness of 463 dead organ donors and their family members, 1270 Australian lives would be saved by organ transplants in 2020.

- 14,352 patients have got transplantation from 5029 dead organ donors since the programme began in 2009.

Between 2009 and 2018, Canada's dead donation rate increased by 42 percent, despite the fact that the quantity of people who have donated organs after they have died decreased by 41 in 2018 similar to 2017, the number of deceased donors, per million people grew from 14.5 to 20.6. (pmp),resulting In 2009, there were 487 dead donors, and in 2018, there were 762 dead donors. The quantity of dead organ donors has increased at the fastest rate since 2013. Despite the fact that Canada's average number of transplanted organs is lower, Up to 8 organs can be obtained from a solo dead donor [14].

7. India

Organ donation is permitted under INDIAN law. The NDTV-Fortis more to give campaign is aimed at increasing organ donation awareness. Organ shortages claim the lives of 5 million people per year. Just 1000 people with liver diseases receive a liver transplant. 2, 20,000 people are waiting for kidney transplants, but only 15,000 are successful. Why INDIA needs to donate organs: -People waiting for corneal The number of transplants is in the tens of thousands, while the There are also tens of thousands of people waiting for heart transplants. People in need of lung transplants: 20,000.

Among the In India, The group of individuals who require organ transplants vs. the amount of organs that are available is vastly different. Around 1.8 lakh people are reported to be affected by renal failure, but only 6000 renal Every year, thousands of transplants are performed. An approximate 2 lac have been identified with end-stage renal disease as a result of cancer, with only 10–15% of them saved by a timely liver transplant. As a result, India needs approximately 25–30 thousand liver transplants each year, but only about 1500 are performed. Per year, 10 to 15 heart transplants are performed in India, despite the fact that 50,000 people die of heart failure each year. Every year, 25,000 cornea transplants are performed against a demand of 1 lakh.

Between 2013 and 2018, India reported 49,155 transplants, including 39,000 There were 10,155 surviving organ receivers and 10,155 dead organ recipients. Organs donated included kidneys (32,584, dead donor = 5748), The liver (6416, deceased donation = 2967), heart (895, deceased donation = 895), lung (459, dead donation = 459), pancreas (78, dead donation = 78), and small intestine (dead donor = 8) were all transplanted. As per information from 2018, In terms of overall transplantation, India was the making it the second largest transplanting nation. The current state of dead donor organ transplants, as well as its obstacles and remedies are discussed in this article [15].

The health-care system at the district is a top half organization that acts as a link among state and regional systems mostly on one hand, and networks in the periphery on another like PHC and sub-centers on the other. It gathers data at the state level and adapts it to local needs before sending it out to the periphery. As a result, it assumes the position of a manager and raises a slew of general, operational, and administrative questions about health-care management. The district official with ultimate authority is the District Medical and Health Officer is another name for the Chief Medical and Health Officer is the person in charge of the medical and health aspects of the health and family care programmes are overseen by these officer in the district and are also DMOs and CMOs are two terms for the same thing. They are responsible for carrying out programmes in accordance with policies developed and finalized at the state and federal levels.

The In rural areas, sick people and others who have particular complaints or who have been referred by As their first point of contact with a licensed public sector doctor, Primary Health Centres are sub-centers for curative, preventive, and promotional health care. In hilly, tribal, or challenging areas, a typical Primary Health Centre with 4–6 indoor/observation beds serves. The city has a population of 20,000 inhabitants, while the plains have a population of 30,000. It serves as a referral center for six sub-centers, sending patients to the In the sub-district and district, there are Higher-order public hospitals and Community Health Centers (30-bed hospitals).

In India, the idea of a Primary Health Centre (PHC) is not new. The Bhore Committee proposed the PHC as a basic health unit in 1946, along with goal of supplying rural residents with comprehensive effective therapeutic and protective healthcare as close to the people as possible.

Indian health planners imagine as the proper structure for delivering medical facilities to the village community, PHC and its Sub-Centres (SCs) should be used. PHCs should be formed in community development blocks to render comprehensive medical care to population in remote areas, according to The 1st conference of the Central Council of Health was held in January 1953.

These clinics serve as outlying health-care organizations with almost no involvement from the communities. These centers have been increasingly criticized for not being able to offer sufficient health care, in part because they are understaffed, underequipped, and lacking basic facilities.

It was proposed that the PHCs be reorganized to provide more efficient coverage. According to the 6th 5 Year Plan, one PHC per 30, thousands remote area communities one PHC per 20,000 in the lowland residents in mountainous, regional, and underdeveloped areas (1983–1988). The United States has founded 23,109 Primary Health Care Centers (PHCs) since that time (In September of 2004).

Primary care clinics (PHCs) are the backbone of villages healthcare institutions, serving as the first point of contact for those who are unwell and are sent to sub-centers for healing, protective, and promotional medical care. Six sub-centers use it as a referral center, sending patients to the appropriate location. There are Community Health Centres (30-bed hospitals) and higher-level services available at the sub-district and district levels, but no public hospitals. There are 4–6 indoor beds reserved for patients.

In a number of rural dispensaries, PHCs have been created. A PHC has a Medical Officer on board, as well as 14 paramedical and other personnel. The country had 22, 370 PHCs in use as of March 2007. A medical officer, two male and female health assistants, as well as health workers and support staff, are assigned to each PHC. State governments formulate and sustain PHCs as part of the Basic Minimum Services Programme /Minimum Needs Programme, which aims to improve preventive and promotional aspects of healthcare.

8. Methodology

The study adopted pre-experimental research design. This involved Health Workers Working at Primary Health Centers of Pune District. Questionnaires were used as data collection technique. A work site research was conducted among 405 health workers working at primary health center. Probability sampling technique was used for selection of health workers as samples.

Consisting of assessing the existing knowledge and attitude of health workers regarding organ donation. The pretest was administered to 405 samples by using self-administered structured questionnaire. Based on the eligibility criteria, after obtained informed consent from the health workers they have been recruited to intervention by using simple random technique. Assessed the understanding and mindset of health professionals on organ donation by employing standardized questionnaires that are self-administered after the 7 days of intervention.

9. Result

Result shows that, 46.7% of the health workers had poor knowledge (score 0–8), 53.3% of them had average knowledge (score 9–17). In posttest, 6.7% of the health workers had poor knowledge (score 0–8), 49.1% of them had average knowledge (score 9–17) and 44.2% of them had good knowledge (score 18–25) regarding organ donation. This shows that after short film and information booklet, there is remarkable improvement in the knowledge of the health workers regarding organ donation. As health workers got continuous education about various health related information it will be defiantly helpful for gross route level health sectors as well as it will be useful for community people for their promotive, preventive and curative health aspect also.

10. Conclusion

In India, the general population is unaware of the benefits of organ donation for patients and their families. The maximum number of people required are in their twenties and thirties. As a result, receiving a transplant can prevent an entire family from becoming overcrowded.

As problems are existing different measures also carried out to overcome the problem such as improving knowledge and attitude by providing health teaching to people through health workers. Availability of the facility for diagnosing brain death and organ retrieval and transplantation. Legal measures are also adopted by different countries to avoid organ scam and fraud. Research after going through all this thought it will be beneficial if we provide knowledge to the community people not only from urban but also rural area. And the comparison will help to understand the area which is having poor knowledge and required more emphasize. Since health workers are the mediators in rural India, the researchers intended to educate health workers concerning the significance of organ donation. Therefore, the researcher selected the health workers as a sample. Health workers can make a change in the rural public mindset and motivate people to do organ donation for the needy one. Health workers are more close to the general public. They are the one to whom people are sharing their common thoughts, their health issues. As a confident health workers will provide a good suggestions as well as equitable distribution of care to the rural people which improve the health of the public. As a familiar in the rural area health worker can give adequate knowledge about organ donation so that public attitude related organ donation can be change. When public attitude will get change in rural area that will encourage to do organ donation which lead to saves person life.

Les Brown said, "You should be researcher to be teacher, if you don't able to research then you will be not able to teach". This old proverb had always inspired me to move ahead and explore. I had personally experienced while working in the clinical setting as well as I have seen patients waiting for a donor and many times they die waiting for an organ donor. I always wonder why in spite of appraising the importance and need people taking step back. This forced me to take up this topic and to search the root causes other than emotional attachment or pain of losing. At the end, as a community health nurse I found that lack of awareness and false beliefs among the community pulling them back. As community health workers are the working close with community. They understand the community people's point of views. Health workers are the key factors to change the community people's attitude. Hence teaching them can bring a new ray of light in their life especially adults and will help to develop a positive attitude towards organ donation through health workers.

Author details

Mangesh Jabade
Symbiosis College of Nursing, Symbiosis International (Deemed University), Pune, India

*Address all correspondence to: mangesh@scon.edu.in

References

[1] Bezinover D, Saner F. Organ transplantation in the modern era. BMC Anesthesiology. 2019;**19**(1):1-4

[2] Job K, Antony A. Organ donation and transplantation: "Life after Death". Organ Donation and Transplantation: Current Status and Future Challenges. 2018:17

[3] Shroff S. Legal and ethical aspects of organ donation and transplantation. Indian Journal of Urology. 2009;**25**(3):348

[4] Nöhre M, Schieffer E, Hanke A, Pape L, Schiffer L, Schiffer M, et al. Obesity after kidney transplantation - Results of a KTx360° substudy. Frontiers in Psychiatry. 2020;**11**:399

[5] Organ_transplantation @ en.wikipedia.org. (n.d.). Available from: https://en.wikipedia.org/wiki/Organ_transplantation

[6] Statistics @ Www.Organdonor.Gov. (n.d.). Available from: https://www.organdonor.gov/statistics-stories/statistics.html

[7] Tilney NL. Transplant: From Myth to Reality. Yale University Press; 2003

[8] Abouna GM, Barabas AZ, Alexander F, Boyd N, Todd JK, Kinniburgh DW, et al. Animal models of hepatic failure for evaluation of artificial liver support techniques. In: Artificial Organs. London: Palgrave; 1977. pp. 351-362

[9] In 1977 The SEOPF launched The United Network for Organ Sharing (UNOS) is a 501(c)(3) non-profit organisation that pioneered computer-assisted organ matching. programme of its kind (UNOS)

[10] The year 2014 marks the first time that a successful uterus transplant has resulted in a live birth (Sweden)

[11] Murray JE. Human organ transplantation: Background and consequences. Science. 1992;**256**(5062): 1411-1416

[12] Savoia P. Gaspare Tagliacozzi and Early Modern Surgery: Faces, Men, and Pain. Routledge; 2019

[13] Massey EK, Ambagtsheer F, Weimar W, editors. Ethical, Legal and Psychosocial Aspects of Transplantation: Global Challenges. Lengerich: Pabst Science Publishers; 2017

[14] Kute V, Ramesh V, Shroff S, Guleria S, Prakash J. Deceased-donor organ transplantation in India: Current status, challenges, and solutions. Experimental and Clinical Transplantation. 2020;**18**(Suppl 2):31-42

[15] Donation-myths-facts @ www.organdonor.gov. (n.d.). Available from: https://www.organdonor.gov/about/facts-terms/donation-myths-facts.html

Chapter 5

Accommodating Individual Differences: Tailored Messages to Improve the Effectiveness of Message Delivery for Self-Management of Chronic Diseases

Kyung Jung Han

Abstract

User-generated content and platforms on personal health management through apps are commonly used these days as individuals can share their information with others and customize the platform of any media or software/website by their information gathering patterns. For example, a 7-year-old boy familiar with YouTube may view some subscribed channels to learn more about the gummy bear vitamin he takes daily. However, an 80-year-old woman may have trouble gathering information about the 50+ women's vitamin products and whether it is okay to take them without conflicting with her current health condition, unless she calls her health providers or visits a local pharmacy directly. Likewise, this chapter will further discuss the effectiveness of individual behavioral changes by tailored messages with individual differences. An experimental study will be introduced, exploring individual differences to examine health messages. Ultimately, with differences in value orientation, we can consider constructing individualized or tailored health messages. Therefore, more effective ways of creating tailored health messages for technology-based health management interventions will be considered, helping self-management of chronic diseases.

Keywords: health management intervention (HMI), chronic diseases, psychological reactance, health literacy, experiment

1. Introduction

Health literacy matters when an individual is involved in health management intervention (HMI). In the HMI program, intervention users can receive general and individualized health information, set personal goals, self-management, and physical activity or diet goals, and monitor their health conditions [1]. Although the users do not communicate with health professionals daily, they can still check and report their health conditions. The HMI program can offer an extended reach to the users through health education, self-care support, and facilitated communication between intervention users or between intervention users and health care providers [2].

In terms of strategic communication, professional communicators and scholars are focused on developing health messages released in HMIs. Readers perceive the same health information differently depending on how health messages are tailored. Since individuals receive personalized or tailored health messages highlighting specific information, readers become more or less interested in the issue. In other words, because individuals have different values and perspectives on the same information and form different opinions after getting the information, tailored messages are more effective in getting readers' attention. Thus, tailored messages are created to accommodate the individual perspectives of readers, considering individual differences in personal interests, concerns, and need for information [3].

However, there are also barriers to bringing about positive behavior changes. When one feels that something interrupts one's autonomy or freewill, one is likely to reject what an external subject has encouraged one to change. In this study, value orientation and reactance theory will be leading principles. They will be applied to explore a dynamic of attitudinal and behavioral decision-making processes.

An experimental study will examine purpose in life and behavioral intention for healthy behavior change. Applying this life-based knowledge, the current study empirically seeks to prove key elements promoting and impeding healthy behaviors. A study introduced in this chapter will also focus on finding useful elements to include in informative or persuasive health messages to help readers absorb the delivered information more effectively and comply with suggested behaviors. The context of this study is technology-based HMIs delivering tailored or individualized health messages promoting healthy behavior changes. Specifically, healthy behavior changes reducing risk factors of diabetes will be highlighted for creating effective health messages in this study.

1.1 Message tailoring for health literacy associated with individual differences

Patient-centered communication (PCC) is a communicational approach that considers the needs and desires of the patient [4]. PCC improves patient satisfaction and behavioral outcomes [4, 5]. In other words, patients' values, needs, and goals are taken seriously to build better relationships and lead patients to make better decisions [6, 7]. Because the health professional is the initial source of health information, the health professional's communication skill influences the patient's adherence to follow suggested guidance [8]. Thus, PCC uses strategic techniques such as involving the patient in the discussion, exploring the patient's ideas and concerns, and caring about the patient's understanding [9, 10].

Previous studies [11, 12] proved that message tailoring strategies associate with different levels of health literacy in patients. In reference [11], customized HMIs had better self-management outcomes for type 2 diabetes management, such as physical activity, quality of life, and diabetes knowledge. Besides, [12] emphasized the importance of mutual understanding between health providers and patients as they tested the effectiveness of tailored/universal language use for patients with high/low health literacy. The result showed that low health literacy patients had a better understanding when physicians interacted with tailored languages. Such findings support a patient-centered approach to developing health messages with a clear understanding of individuals' needs, interests, and health literacy.

This chapter considers individuals' value orientation as a promising variable for customizing health messages. Vic Strecher introduced personal value orientation as an essential category for tailoring messages, a leading researcher and digital innovator in tailored messaging. His book *On Purpose* [See 13] made a compelling case for personal value orientations as a critical determinant of healthy behavior changes. Considering one's life purpose, self-directed, positive change is possible [13]. As a health professional, he found a pivotal linkage between purpose in life and health behavior changes. It shows the importance of knowing and recalling one's purpose in life when one encounters difficulty in decision-making. Specifically, one's life purpose can be a useful element for promoting healthy behaviors.

1.2 Health management interventions (HMIs) for diabetes

Many studies on technology-based diabetes HMIs have been conducted to improve the effectiveness of target behavior changes [14–16]. As participants receive health information regularly and check their health condition during a specific period (e.g. 3, 6, or 12 months), their target behaviors have been tracked through involved interventions. The major measurements to assess the effectiveness of interventions include HbA_{1c} [17], BMI [18, 19], physical activity [20, 21], and self-efficacy [22].

Generally, health care practitioners and researchers expect technology driven solutions to provide various benefits, such as improving patient outcomes and saving health care fees. However, there are few empirically homogeneous studies, including the same type of technologies or interventions and showing significant effects of the intervention on behavior changes [14, 15]. Even though there are some significant effects on target behavior changes, standard features of interventions leading to healthy behavior changes cannot easily be found due to a lack of standardized protocols and suggested variables considered in the intervention design process. Such heuristic conclusions require health program developers and researchers to consider a more comprehensive approach to various strategies and technologies for intervention development.

In terms of the effect of health messages, many variables need to be considered in the message development stage. Some variables can be facilitators for following the guideline of the health messages, but others can be barriers to compliance with the suggestion of the messages. Some influencers of individual decision-making are individual values (e.g. desired consequences of healthy behavior change), personal beliefs (e.g. expected outcomes, acceptability, and self-efficacy), and previous knowledge, among others [23]. When individuals receive tailored materials implementing those influencers, individuals reveal more (a) positive thoughts about the provided materials, (b) thoughts reflecting a personal connection to the materials, (c) thoughts indicating that a self-assessment took place, and (d) intentions to make behavioral changes [3]. In other words, having an informative focus on health messages is not enough to have expected effects on health message readers. Instead, influencers triggering individuals' evaluation of or interest in the news should be carefully considered. Thus, the study introduced in this chapter sheds light on the influencers of individual decision-making when individuals receive health messages, including suggestions for healthy behavior changes. Specifically, individual value orientations determining life purpose and psychological reactance preventing healthy behavior changes are the focus of this study.

There are gaps in the linkage between individual influencers and message effects, as shown by individual attitude and source appraisal toward the suggested behaviors and messages and ultimate behavior changes. Specifically, the interaction of health messages and personal value orientation as a stimulator of recalling individual life purpose and complying with suggested behavior changes needs to be studied further for the following reasons.

First, the studies on intervention programs for health education and healthy behavior changes have not much focused on developing strategic messages. The distinction between general and individualized information [1] is a sort of effort to consider differences in message development, but it is not enough. Most previous studies targeting healthy behavior changes via intervention programs [14–16] are more focused on the relationship between outcome measurement and functional features (e.g. monitoring, goal setting, peer chatting, personal challenges, etc.) and modality of interventions (e.g. website, email, phone call, app tracking, etc.). These are important, but it is not enough to encompass the overall effectiveness of interventions. The correlation between individualized messages and intervention effects must be considered more closely.

Furthermore, individual value orientations determining purpose in life have not been proved statistically as a precondition of behavioral intentions [16]. Although scholars have tried to link the presence and absence of personal value orientation and consistency and inconsistency between value orientation and suggested behavior change [24], these ideas must be further explored.

1.3 Projected behavioral changes by HMIs

Personal value orientation has been considered an essential influencer of healthy behavior changes. A healthy lifestyle is one of the fundamental health promotion goals. As for highlighting health and linking it to personal value orientation, people are affected by the value and perform the health-promoting behaviors [25]. Values are used as a starting point to decide on meaningful activities and increase the likelihood that when the activities are matched to the values, individuals will reach their goals [26]. Indeed, values are linked to individual health behaviors and are used for health education [27].

In previous studies, personal value orientation has been utilized for positive health behavior changes [26, 27]. For example, as a reinforcer that maintains and strengthens depression control, personal value orientation was used for depression management. In encouraging healthy behavior change, establishing values helps individuals ensure that selected healthy behaviors will have positive effects over time. Instead of being random required to choose a healthy behavior, connecting it to values positively impacts achieving ultimate behavioral goals [27]. Additionally, people who received inductive messages intended to raise self-enhancement value rated that they are at higher risk for HIV and showed higher intention to purchase condoms and to take education programs than people who did not receive self-enhancement messages [28]. As an element of message tailoring, discounts can be directly reflected to help one accomplish one's own goal in the self-management of diabetes.

Psychological reactance can be examined to measure behavioral changes by tailored messages with a personal value orientation. Reference [29] introduced psychological reactance theory (PRT) as a framework explaining the rejection of persuasive messages with several variables (intention to comply with suggested behaviors, source appraisal, etc.). In other words, PRT describes possible reasons for noncompliance with recommended behaviors [30]. It is important to project whether patients or intervention participants will comply with the suggested behavioral changes or not. It connects to their satisfaction with tailored messages. Reactance is a sort of voluntary motivation against external pressure caused by intrinsic motivation. Reactant individuals are likely to show negative attitudes [31]. In this study, the meaning of attitude is closer to affective and cognitive attitude rather than conative attitude, because the behavioral intention is separately measured. In particular, the attitude toward the suggested health behavior and attitude toward the health messages are the variables measured in this study.

2. Hypotheses

Although personal value orientation is positively applied to healthy behavior changes [25, 27], few studies connect personal value orientation to psychological reactance. However, it is not difficult to discern the relevance of unique value orientation and psychological reactance if "self" and "the subject of control" are considered. When healthy behavior changes are promoted, personal value orientation relates to the things vital to one's life [27]. Thinking about one's value orientation is to reflect on oneself and one's life. In doing so, self-identity is ensured and helps select healthy behaviors [26]. In contrast, psychological reactance is caused by eliminating one's freedom. That is, reactance is caused by threatening one's self-esteem [32].

Although thinking about oneself is equal to both personal value orientation and reactance, reactance has a negative effect on compliance with suggested behavior changes [33]. Once reactance is aroused, reactant individuals tend to be autonomous and dominant [34]. This implies that there may be a counterpart effect of reactance in triggering personal value orientation for healthy behavior changes or for complying with suggested behaviors.

Reactance is aroused differently depending on individual characteristics. Certain situations appear to arouse more reactance than others; certain people seem more reactant than others [34]. In other words, individuals likely evaluate the same health message on diabetes differently depending on individual differences and given conditions or messages. In this study, differences in personal value orientation can be a cue to determine the degree of reactance arousal.

Additionally, there is a difference in the meaning of two extreme personal value orientations: self-enhancement and self-transcendence. For self-enhancement, the nature of control is internal to oneself [35]; for self-transcendence, the nature of control is external. Thus, people who have more self-enhancement values are likely to be more sensitive to having their autonomy threatened. Although narcissism is the extreme case when self-enhancement value is overloaded, we can also find a cue explaining the relationship between self-enhancement and reactance: "Narcissists have an inflated sense of entitlement, so they should be more prone to reactance because they are more likely than others to believe they deserve things that they are not getting" [36]. It has been shown that narcissists react more than others [37]. For self-enhancement value, it is uncertain how much reactance is aroused for those who value self-enhancement in their life. Still, at least the difference between self-enhancement and self-transcendence values is likely to be disclosed.

> *H1. Triggering personal value orientation will be associated with psychological reactance.*

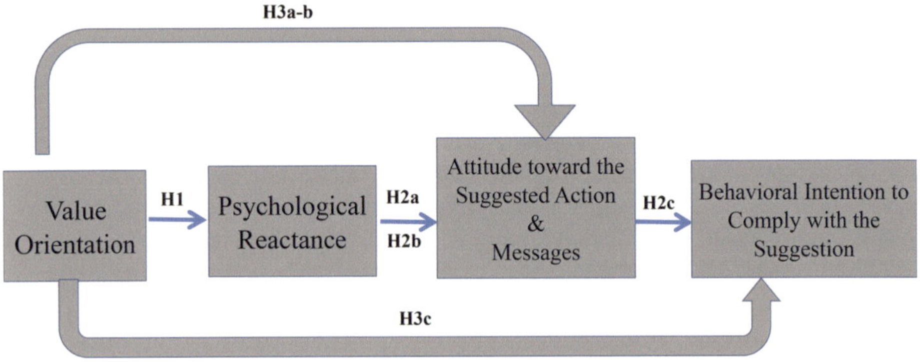

Figure 1.
Hypotheses.

> *H1a. Participants whose self-enhancement value is triggered will show higher psychological reactance than those whose self-transcendence value is triggered.*

Regarding health behavior change, high reactant patients are less likely to follow a suggested behavior (e.g. smoking or drinking cessation); low reactant patients are more likely to follow a suggested behavior [33].

> *H2. Psychological reactance will be negatively associated with a) attitude toward a suggested behavior, b) attitude toward the presented message, and c) behavioral intention to change.*

To promote health behavior change, triggering personal value orientation could give more control over the determinants of one's life. A previous study tested the relationship triggering personal value orientation and behavioral outcomes. The study found that a participant who received a message triggering personal value orientation could link health behavior with ultimate consequences and felt more control over their behavior [28]. Recalling personal value orientation leads one to think more critically about one's behavior and exert more control over one's behavior. Triggering personal value orientation improves one's ability to link the value to decision-making and increases a specific behavioral intention (**Figure 1**) [28].

> *H3. Triggering personal value orientation will be associated with a) a more negative attitude toward a suggested behavior, b) a more negative attitude toward the presented message, and c) higher behavioral intention.*

3. Methodology

Participants. This study has two main criteria for participation: age and diabetes. For age, participants between the ages of 45 and 64 years are recruited through *Amazon Mechanical Turk* (https://www.mturk.com/mturk/welcome). The researcher opened a HIT or project on MTurk with two keywords of the study: experiment and news article evaluation. Participants signed up to the study to evaluate health-related news articles possibly released in health intervention programs. As participants initiated the experiment, they were told about a more detailed summary of the study through an informed consent form. Participants granted their agreement to participate in the study.

They are in the mid-aged adults. A priori G*Power analysis was conducted for the expected effect size of .25 with an α = .05. The study revealed that a sample size of 232 was needed to sufficiently power the design test.

Procedures. Personal value orientation is tested in advance before presenting health-related intervention messages. Self-enhancement or self-transcendence value is categorized to consider individual differences in value orientation. Then, both groups of participants are given two health-related articles: physical activity and health nutrition. One condition was randomly assigned among a selected set of stimuli (N = 2). For example, if one evaluates self-enhancement value higher in questions about personal value orientation included in the recruitment survey, they are randomly assigned to one of two self-enhancement value conditions (1: self-enhancement-presence; 2: self-enhancement-absence). It applies to the self-transcendence group.

Personal Value Orientation. In this study, value orientation is operationally defined by the value orientation in Value Theory [35], because personal value orientation shows the most important element in one's life. It has the power to move one's mind. Among many value orientations, this study selected the two most extreme value orientations: self-enhancement and self-transcendence. Personal value orientation is a facilitator of healthy behavior changes. It is measured whether self-enhancement or self-transcendence value drives your purpose in life. Depending on individual value orientation, participants receive one of four conditions triggering either self-enhancement or self-transcendence value for promoting healthy behavior changes. Self-enhancement and self-transcendence values are measured using 20 items (self-enhancement, n = 4, α = .834; self-transcendence, n = 16, α = .907) with a Likert scale of −1 (*opposed to my values*) and 0 (*not important*) to 7 (*extremely important*). Eight items are a value orientation measurement [38], such as "social power" and "wealth" for self-enhancement value and "equality" and "a world at peace" for self-transcendence value; the other 12 items are drawn from *On Purposes* [13 , pp.73], such as "popularity" and "admiration" for self-enhancement value and "empathy" and "compassion" for self-transcendence value.

Stimuli. Two news articles were from a real online daily news outlet, *Healthday* (http://healthday.com). "Diabetes" was used as a search term for news articles, and the two articles were selected considering news frames and article-released dates. One article on health nutrition management and the other one on active physical exercise were presented to participants. Both articles were written in the typical form of news articles with a headline, subhead, journalist's name, day and date, and an accompanying picture, respectively. Based on the original articles, the length of the article's presence/absence of a value orientation was considered for creating stimuli. The number of words was controlled.

Personal value orientation phrases in stimuli. To create messages triggering personal value orientation, concepts of self-enhancement and self-transcendent values are carefully considered [13]. For instance, in the self-enhancement value condition for nutrition management, two sentences were added at the end of the news article: sentence 1. Caring about your health condition is directly linked to caring about your success in your life—sentence 2. Your diet is like saving money; considering your nutrition condition in daily life is a good investment for your life success.

Your diet is like savings; considering your nutrition condition in daily life is a good investment for your family or significant others. In contrast, for the self-transcendence value presence condition for nutrition management, two sentences were added at the end of the news article: Sentence 1. Caring about individuals' health conditions is directly linked to caring about others significant to you or those who need your help during the rest of your life—sentence 2.

3.1 Measured variables

Personal Value Orientation. For manipulation check of unique value orientation, two items are measured: "The information in the news article tried to make me think about my value orientation." and "The information in the news article tried to make me think about changing/continuing my current health behaviors as guided in the news article for my value orientation," with a Likert scale of 7 (*strongly agree*) to 1 (*strongly disagree*).

Psychological Reactance. The state of reactance operationally defines psychological reactance. A four-item stating reactance scale [39, 40] with a Likert scale of 7 (*strongly agree*) to 1 (*strongly disagree*) is measured. For example, the questions in the nutrition management condition are as follows: "I am uncomfortable being told how to feel about managing vitamin D"; "I do not like that I am being told how to feel about managing vitamin D"; "It irritates me that the news article told me how to feel about managing vitamin D"; and "I dislike that I am being told how to feel about managing vitamin D." Reliability analysis confirmed its internal consistency (α = .937).

Attitude toward Suggested Behaviors. Attitude toward suggested behaviors is operationally defined by evaluating personal attitude toward suggested behaviors: vitamin D management and physical activity. Participants' attitude toward the suggested behaviors was asked through seven-point semantic differential questions [31]. The main question is, "Based on this information, how would you rate your attitude toward vitamin D management/exercise?" The word pairs used are negative/positive, unnecessary/necessary, good/bad (reverse coded), foolish/wise, detrimental/beneficial, and favorable/unfavorable (reserve coded). Reliability analysis confirmed its internal consistency (α = .929).

Attitude toward Presented Health Messages. Attitude toward presented health messages is operationally defined by the personal impression of the presented health message. Three items gauged participants' attitudes toward the health message. A set of seven-point semantic differential scales is anchored by bad/good, favorable/unfavorable (reverse-coded), and negative/positive [32, 41], as the answer to "How would you rate your overall impression of this information on the following scale?" Reliability analysis confirmed its internal consistency (α = .807).

Behavioral Intention to Comply with Suggested Behaviors. Behavioral intention to comply with suggested behaviors is operationally defined by the willingness to conform to the suggested behavior. A 100-point rating scale is used for measuring respondents' behavioral intention. A single item is asked: "How willing are you to manage vitamin D or exercise regularly in the following week?" [31, 39]. Reliability analysis confirmed its internal consistency (α = .807).

4. Results of experiment study

Tests of Hypotheses. H1 predicted that triggering individual value orientation or how much my life is worth to me would be associated with psychological reactance. A one-way ANOVA was used to examine the level of psychological reactance to the presence and absence of triggering personal value orientation. For the nutrition article, the analysis also showed a significant difference in psychological reactance between triggering personal value orientation and not triggering personal value orientation, $F(1,309) = 167.01, p = .000, \eta_p^2 = 0.35$. That is, those who read a nutrition-related article triggering personal value orientation have lower psychological reactance than others who read another article not triggering personal value orientation. For the physical activity article, the analysis also showed a significant difference in psychological reactance between triggering personal value orientation and not triggering personal value orientation, $F(1,309) = 71.30$, p = .000, $\eta_p^2 = 0.19$. That is, those who read a physical activity-related article triggering personal value orientation have lower psychological reactance than others who read another article not triggering personal value orientation. Thus, H1 was supported.

With H1, one with a self-enhancement value was expected to show higher psychological reactance than the other with a self-transcendence value (H1a).

For the article on nutrition, the result of a one-way ANOVA revealed a significant difference in psychological reactance by individual value orientation, $F(1,155) = 79.40, p = .000, \eta_p^2 = .34$. Those with more self-enhancement values showed higher psychological reactance than others with more self-transcendence values. For the article on physical activity, the result of a one-way ANOVA showed a significant difference in psychological reactance by individual value orientation, $F(1,160) = 85.33$, p = .000, $\eta_p^2 = .35$. Those with more self-enhancement values showed higher psychological reactance than others with more self-transcendence values. Thus, H1a was supported.

Psychological reactance was associated with some of the dependent variables. Particularly for nutrition, psychological reactance was positively associated with attitude toward the presented message ($F[1, 309] = .16$, p = .048). However, attitude toward the presented message was expected to relate to psychological reactance negatively. Additionally, other variables were negatively correlated, but they were not significant.

For physical activity, psychological reactance was negatively associated with attitude toward the presented message ($F[1, 309] = 11.90$, p = .001), attitude toward a suggested behavior ($F[1, 309] = 19.42$, p = .000), and behavioral intention to follow a suggested behavior ($F[1, 309] = 4.56$, p = .033). In terms of correlation, these results show that higher psychological reactance is associated with a negative attitude toward the presented message ($\beta = -.17$), a negative attitude toward a suggested behavior ($\beta = -.18$), and a lower behavior intention to follow a suggested behavior ($\beta = -.11$). H2 was partially supported.

For H3 test, on the nutrition-related article, triggering self-enhancement value was significantly associated with a) more negative attitude toward a suggested behavior than self-transcendence value, M_self-enhancement = 5.62 (SD = 1.09), N = 68; M_self-transcendence = 6.06 (SD = 1.26), N = 89; F(1,155) = 5.39, p = .02, ηp2 = .03. Thus, H3 was partially supported.

5. Discussion

This study aimed to consider how tailored messages as a part of technology-based interventions could become more effective in helping self-management to relieve diabetes symptoms. This study was guided by the idea that strategic health messages that consider facilitators and barriers work differently even though they include the same information. An individual value orientation was regarded as a facilitator of suggested healthy behavior change and freedom threat as a barrier to suggested healthy behavior change. Specifically, a personal value orientation or how my life has worth for me was represented by different value orientations such as self-enhancement value and self-transcendence value. To develop these ideas further, earlier literature was reviewed in terms of (1) patient-centered message strategies considering tailored messages according to individual features such as personal value orientation, (2) psychological reactance theory as a barrier to suggested healthy behavior change, and (3) potential integration effects of message strategies and psychological reactance.

With such ideas, an experimental study was conducted to measure levels of psychological reactance caused by freedom threat, motivation to restore threatened freedom, attitude to the suggested healthy behaviors/messages, intention to comply with suggestions, and source appraisal. To do this, participants in the study were presented with two news articles on nutrition and physical activity to repeat identically manipulated tests for one of among eight conditions: 4 (personal value orientation—self-enhancement value: presence vs. absence; self-transcendence value: presence vs. absence) x 2 (freedom threat: presence vs. absence) between subjects for adults with diabetes.

The data indicate that a facilitator of behavior change—personal value orientation—and a barrier to it—freedom threat—affect decision-making against suggested behavior. Specifically, triggering personal value orientation and freedom threat was associated with psychological reactance. Psychological reactance was mainly associated with higher motivation to restore threatened freedom, a more negative attitude toward a suggested behavior and the presented message, lower behavioral intention, and lower source appraisal (dependent variables). There were correlations between dependent variables of psychological reactance. Psychological reactance is also mediated between personal value orientation and some dependent variables (i.e. motivation to restore suggested behavior and attitude toward a suggested behavior). However, no interaction effect between personal value orientation and freedom threat was found for psychological reactance on physical activity and all dependent variables. Direct relationships between personal value orientation and dependent variables were also not found.

Summary of Findings. The following section of this chapter interprets the research findings. It discusses practical and theoretical implications for designing strategic health messages and developing related theories: value theory and psychological reactance theory. First, results regarding the direct effect of a facilitator and a barrier on psychological reactance are discussed. It is valuable to apply for designing mediated intervention programs, since certain factors can be a booster (personal value orientation) or a barrier (psychological reactance). Considering individuals' response patterns can help finding actual effects. In this study, a discussion of the direct effect follows this: 1) the direct effect of psychological reactance to dependent variables related to decision-making; 2) the direct effect of personal value orientation on dependent variables; 3) correlation between dependent variables, and 4) direct interaction effect of freedom threat on dependent variables. Finally, the mediation effect of psychological reactance between personal value orientation and dependent variables is examined.

The direct effect of a facilitator and a barrier to continue an intervention. The first hypothesis predicted that triggering personal value orientation would be associated with psychological reactance. In terms of value orientation, it was predicted that participants whose self-enhancement value was triggered would show higher psychological reactance than other participants whose self-transcendence was triggered. The hypothesis was supported on all counts. Participants reported that they had lower psychological reactance when they read value-triggering articles. This result shows that personal value orientation attenuates psychological reactance. The concepts—personal value orientation and psychological reactance—both focus on "self," so it is not difficult to link these, although previous studies have not tested this linkage. Personal value orientation reflects oneself and one's life [27]. In contrast, reactance is a negative response when one recognizes that one's self-esteem is threatened [32]. Thus, H1 proved that when one reads health-related news, if the author approaches readers in terms of a personal value orientation or primary value in one's life, the negative effect of psychological reactance is attenuated.

Additionally, H1a considered different value orientations: self-enhancement and self-transcendence. As predicted, the result revealed that participants who read a self-enhancement value-triggering article showed higher psychological reactance than others who read a self-transcendence value-triggering article. H1a was supported. In terms of psychological reactance, if reactance is aroused, one tends to be dominant and autonomous [34]. Similarly, if one thinks self-enhancement value is important, it is likely for one to have a locus of control internal to oneself [35]. Thus, although triggering personal value orientation attenuates psychological reactance, self-enhancement value remains more of an effect of psychological reactance than self-transcendence, whose locus of control is external (influenced by external situations). As a newly tested variable attenuating psychological reactance, triggering a personal value orientation opens a possibility applicable to strategic health messages. However, different individual value orientations should be considered simultaneously, because triggering value produces other effects depending on individual value orientation. As a representative example, this study examined two extreme value orientations: self-enhancement and self-transcendence. H1a proved that triggering personal value orientation is more effective for participants with self-transcendence values.

Direct effect on decision-making for a suggested behavior in an intervention. The second and third hypotheses predicted an immediate impact on dependent variables related to decision-making (i.e. attitude toward a suggested behavior, attitude toward the presented message, and behavioral intention to comply with suggested behavior). Specifically, H2 considered the direct effect of psychological reactance on dependent variables. The direct impact of psychological reactance was significant for motivation to restore freedom and attitude toward the presented messages for the nutrition article. On the other hand, the direct effect of psychological reactance was significant for all dependent variables for the physical activity article. The partial acceptance of H3 strengthened the previous result of the psychological reactance theory [29, 31]. This result proved that psychological reactance was associated with consequential decision-making for suggested behavior changes. It shows how important control for psychological reactance is. To achieve expected outcomes, health communication strategists should not ignore the negative effect of causing psychological reactance so that readers reject the suggested behavior with negative attitudes, higher motivation to restore freedom, and derogation of the source. However, the message topic is still worth considering here because not all topics resulted in the same outcomes.

H3 predicted the direct effect of personal value orientation on dependent variables related to decision-making. The result was not significant, so the hypothesis was not supported. Referring to H1, which considered the different types of value orientations together, alternative H3 was analyzed. The direct effect of different value orientations on dependent variables was partially significant. Specifically, triggering self-enhancement value was significantly associated with attitude toward a suggested behavior for nutrition, and it was significantly associated with motivation to restore threatened freedom for physical activity. There are many perspectives to be considered to succeed in developing effective health messages using personal value orientations. However, previous studies that evaluated health contexts with the most important value in one's life showed the positive effect of this variable on positive behavior changes [24]. This suggests that other mediators or moderators may affect decision-making when one's primary personal value orientation is triggered.

Practical Implications. This investigation aimed to find determinants of persuasive message effects, specifically in the context of health news articles helping with diabetes self-management.

This study can help health professionals better understand effective strategies for health message development for diabetes self-management interventions. In particular, this study is different from the previous studies done mainly through health professionals for a similar topic. It investigated means for practitioners to develop effective messages for self-management diabetes intervention in terms of recruitment, retention, and ultimate healthy behavior changes from the perspective of a strategic communication researcher. In other words, the study intended to help practitioners develop different messages for self-management diabetes intervention with the fresh eyes of a strategic communication researcher. Considering a facilitator (i.e. personal value orientation) and a barrier (i.e. freedom threat) to the persuasive effect of messages suggesting healthy behavior changes for people with prediabetes/diabetes, the current study sought to find key elements determining the success or failure of the health-message.

With such an idea, this research provides various angles of implications applicable to an intervention program: 1) development of persuasive messages and determination of necessary baseline information for initial recruitment in a diabetes intervention, 2) development of related and valuable messages for participants to increase retention rates, and 3) ultimately, development of effective messages to facilitate behavior changes in the long term.

Theoretical Implications. The present study expanded the depth and breadth of theory for the following three reasons:

First, this study examined a new variable—personal value orientation—for message tailoring and linked it to the original psychological reactance theory (PRT).

Second, the basic assumptions of the original psychological reactance theory—about reactance—were elaborated and strengthened. That is, the original relationship between variables was retested to examine the interaction between antecedents of reactance and dependent variables of reactance.

Third, the statistical power of existing assumptions had increased alongside the testing significance of the relationship between variables. Although the direct effect was not supported for a behavior change, the direct effect from personal value orientation on psychological reactance was fully funded. It was suggested in previous studies, such as the research of Martin et al. (2011), but this was not thorough enough to support personal value orientation as a pretreatment variable.

Lastly, the interdisciplinary approach (e.g. strategic communication, psychology, information technology, health, etc.) applied in this study worked to match similar studies conducted in different academic areas. This implies fruitful opportunities opened for researchers to collaborate on an intervention development project to help self-management of diabetes symptoms.

Conclusion. The health literacy matters when patients want to care about their health. Considering individuals' different levels of health literacy, other needs and personal values can be counted together. It is to help patients continue their health plans or boost decision-making complying with suggestions by health providers. The COVID-19 response clearly illustrates how inequities can sharpen and deepen when publics did not receive appropriate information to take actions [42]. It does not include adjusting the level of health knowledge or health literacy only, but also it needs to consider how well tailoring health messages for target audiences.

Conflict of interest

The authors declare no conflict of interest.

Author details

Kyung Jung Han
California State University, Bakersfield, USA

*Address all correspondence to: khan1@csub.edu

References

[1] Neve M, Morgan PJ, Jones PR, Collins CE. Effectiveness of web-based interventions in achieving weight loss and weight loss maintenance in overweight and obese adults: A systematic review with meta-analysis. Obesity Reviews. 2010;**11**(4):306-321

[2] Lyles CR, Sarkar U, Osborn C. Getting a technology-based diabetes intervention ready for prime time: A review of usability testing studies. Current Diabetes Reports. 2014;**14**(10):1-12

[3] Kreuter MW, Farrell D, Olevitch L, Brennan L. Tailoring Health Messages: Customizing Communication with Computer Technology. Mahwah, NJ: Lawrence Erlbaum Associates; 2013

[4] Epstein R, Street RL. Patient-centered Communication in Cancer Care: Promoting Healing and Reducing Suffering. Bethesda, MD: National Cancer Institute, US Department of Health and Human Services, National Institutes of Health; 2007

[5] Wanzer MB, Booth-Butterfield M, Gruber K. Perceptions of health care providers' communication: Relationships between patient-centered communication and satisfaction. Health Communication. 2004;**16**:363-384

[6] Mead N, Bower P. Patient-centredness: A conceptual framework and review of the empirical literature. Social Science & Medicine. 2000;**51**(7):1087-1110

[7] Roter D. The enduring and evolving nature of the patient–physician relationship. Patient Education and Counseling. 2000;**39**(1):5-15

[8] Nair K, Dolovich L, Cassels A, McCormack J, Levine M, Gray J, et al. What patients want to know about their medications: Focus group study of patient and clinician perspectives. Canadian Family Physician. 2002;**48**(1):104-110

[9] Hirsh AT, Atchison JW, Berger JJ, Waxenberg LB, Lafayette-Lucey A, Bulcourf BB, et al. Patient satisfaction with treatment for chronic pain: Predictors and relationship to compliance. The Clinical Journal of Pain. 2005;**21**:302-310

[10] Mast MS, Kindlimann A, Langewitz W. Recipients' perspective on breaking bad news: How you put it really makes a difference. Patient Education and Counseling. 2005;**58**:244-251

[11] Dahal PK, Hosseinzadeh H. Association of health literacy and diabetes self-management: A systematic review. Australian Journal of Primary Health. 2020;**25**:526-533

[12] Schillinger D, Duran ND, McNamara DS, Crossley SA, Balyan R, Karter AJ. Precision communication: Physicians' linguistic adaptation to patients' health literacy. Science. 2021;**17**:eabj2836

[13] Strecher JV. On Purpose: Lessons in Life and Health from the Frog, Dung Beetle, and Julia. Ann Arbor, MI: Dung Beetle Press; 2013

[14] Connelly J, Kirk A, Masthoff J, MacRury S. The use of technology to promote physical activity in Type 2 diabetes management: A systematic review. Diabetic Medicine. 2013;**30**(12): 1420-1432

[15] Free C, Phillips G, Galli L, Watson L, Felix L, Edwards P, et al.

The effectiveness of mobile-health technology-based health behaviour change or disease management interventions for health care consumers: A systematic review. PLoS Medicine. 2013;**10**(1):e1001362

[16] Kelders SM, Kok RN, Ossebaard HC, Van Gemert-Pijnen JE. Persuasive system design does matter: A systematic review of adherence to web-based interventions. Journal of Medical Internet Research. 2012;**14**(6):e152

[17] Lorig K, Ritter PL, Laurent DD, Plant K, Green M, Jernigan VBB, et al. Online diabetes self-management program: A randomized study. Diabetes Care. 2010;**33**(6):1275-1281

[18] Holbrook A, Thabane L, Keshavjee K, Dolovich L, Bernstein B, Chan D, et al. Individualized electronic decision support and reminders to improve diabetes care in the community: COMPETE II randomized trial. Canadian Medical Association Journal. 2009;**181**(1-2):37-44

[19] Glasgow RE, Christiansen SM, Kurz D, King DK, Woolley T, Faber AJ, et al. Engagement in a diabetes self-management website: Usage patterns and generalizability of program use. Journal of Medical Internet Research. 2011;**13**(1):e9. DOI: 10.2196/jmir.1391

[20] Khan MA, Shah S, Grudzien A, Onyejekwe N, Banskota P, Karim S, et al. A diabetes education multimedia program in the waiting room setting. Diabetes Therapy. 2011;**2**(3): 178-188

[21] Richardson J, Letts L, Chan D, Stratford P, Hand C, Price D, et al. Rehabilitation in a primary care setting for persons with chronic illness: A randomized controlled trial. Primary Health Care Research & Development. 2010;**11**(4):382-395. DOI: 10.1017/S1463423610000113

[22] Faridi Z, Liberti L, Shuval K, Northrup V, Ali A, Katz DL. Evaluating the impact of mobile telephone technology on type 2 diabetic patients' self-management: The NICHE pilot study. Journal of Evaluation in Clinical Practice. 2008;**14**(3):465-469

[23] Davis S. Internet-based tailored health communications: Application and future directions. Interface: The Journal of Education, Community and Values. 2007;**7**(3)

[24] Martin RA, MacKinnon S, Johnson J, Rohsenow DJ. Purpose in life predicts treatment outcome among adult cocaine abusers in treatment. Journal of Substance Abuse Treatment. 2011;**40**:183-188

[25] Enjezab B, Farajzadegan Z, Taleghani F, Aflatoonian A. Internal motivations and barriers effective on the healthy lifestyle of middle-aged women: A qualitative approach. Iranian Journal of Nursing and Midwifery Research. 2012;**17**(5):390-398

[26] Largo-Wight E. Identity and value development for a healthy lifestyle. American Journal of Health Education. 2007;**38**(2):104-107

[27] Lejuez CW, Hopko DR, Acierno R, Daughters SB, Pagoto SL. Ten year revision of the brief behavioral activation treatment for depression: Revised treatment manual. Behavior Modification. 2011;**35**(2):111-161

[28] Sherman D, Nelson L, Steele C. Do messages about health risks threaten the self? Increasing the acceptance of threatening health messages via self-affirmation. Personality and Social

Psychology Bulletin. 2000;**26**:1046-1058. DOI: 10.1177/01461672002611003

[29] Brehm JW. A Theory of Psychological Reactance. San Diego, CA: Academic Press; 1966

[30] Quick BL, Stephenson MT. The Reactance Restoration Scale (RRS): A measure of direct and indirect restoration. Communication Research Reports. 2007;**24**(2):131-138

[31] Dillard JP, Shen L. On the nature of reactance and its role in persuasive health communication. Communication Monographs. 2005;**72**:144-168

[32] Goodwin R, Costa P, Adonu J. Social support and its consequences: 'Positive' and 'deficiency' values and their implications for support and self-esteem. The British Journal of Social Psychology. 2004;**43**(3):465-474

[33] Graybar SR, Antonuccio DO, Boutilier LR, Varble DL. Psychological reactance as a factor affecting patient compliance to physician advice. Scandinavian Journal of Behaviour Therapy. 1989;**18**:43-51

[34] Dowd ET. Psychological reactance in health education and promotion. Health Education Journal. 2002;**61**(2):113-124

[35] Schwartz SH. Les valeurs de base de la personne: Théorie, mesures et applications [Basic human values: Theory, measurement, and applications]. Revue Française de Sociologie. 2006;**47**:249-288

[36] Bushman BJ, Bonacci AM, Van Dijk M, Baumeister RF. Narcissism, sexual refusal, and aggression: Testing a narcissistic reactance model of sexual coercion. Journal of Personality and Social Psychology. 2003;**84**(5):1028

[37] Frank SJ, Jackson-Walker S, Marks M, Van-Egeren LA, Loop K, Olson K. From the laboratory to the hospital, adults to adolescents, and disorders to personality: The case of psychological reactance. Journal of Clinical Psychology. 1998;**54**:361-381

[38] De Groot JI, Steg L. Value orientations to explain beliefs related to environmental significant behavior how to measure egoistic, altruistic, and biospheric value orientations. Environment and Behavior. 2008;**40**(3):330-354

[39] Quick BL. What is the best measure of psychological reactance? An empirical test of two measures. Health Communication. 2012;**27**(1):1-9

[40] Lindsey LLM. Anticipated guilt as behavioral motivation: An examination of appeals to help unknown others through bone marrow donation. Human Communication Research. 2005;**31**:453-481

[41] Lafferty BA, Goldsmith RE. Corporate credibility's role in consumers' attitudes and purchase intentions when a high versus a low credibility endorser is used in the ad. Journal of Business Research. 1999;**44**(2):109-116

[42] Jackson DN, Trivedi N, Baur C. Re-prioritizing digital health and health literacy in healthy people 2030 to affect health equity. Health Communication. 2021;**36**(10):1155-1162